Ahmed HARBAOUI

Extradural hematomas of the posterior cerebral fossa

Ahmed HARBAOUI

Extradural hematomas of the posterior cerebral fossa

Diagnosis and treatment

ScienciaScripts

Cover image: www.ingimage.com

This book is a translation from the original published under ISBN 978-620-6-72534-3.

Publisher:
Sciencia Scripts
is a trademark of
Dodo Books Indian Ocean Ltd. and OmniScriptum S.R.L publishing group

120 High Road, East Finchley, London, N2 9ED, United Kingdom
Str. Armeneasca 28/1, office 1, Chisinau MD-2012, Republic of Moldova, Europe
Managing Directors: Ieva Konstantinova, Victoria Ursu
info@omniscriptum.com

Printed at: see last page
ISBN: 978-620-8-35468-8

TABLE OF CONTENTS

INTRODUCTION

Traumatic brain injury (TBI) is a major public health problem in many countries. It is the leading cause of death in the population aged between 15 and 25, and the leading cause of disability before the age of 45 [1].

Extradural haematoma (EDH) or epidural haematoma is an uncommon but potentially serious complication of cranial trauma. It is defined as an accumulation of blood in the epidural space between the internal table of the bone and the dura mater. It represents the neurosurgical emergency par excellence [1].

Locating it in the posterior cerebral fossa is very rare, but is particularly serious as it is most often the result of direct, violent trauma applied directly to the occipital region. The clinical picture is classically defined by a three-stage drama, with the first stage being the trauma, which may be accompanied by an initial loss of consciousness, followed by a period of lucidity or free interval, and then the secondary aggravation phase, in which neurological signs appear, along with an altered state of consciousness [1,2].

The management of extradural haematomas has benefited greatly from advances in medical imaging, and in particular from the advent of cerebral computed tomography (CT), which not only makes it possible to carry out a complete emergency assessment of the lesion, but also to establish the indication for surgery, and to monitor and follow up patients after treatment [2].

In our work, we will study through a retrospective study concerning 25 patients the management of extradural haematomas of the posterior cerebral fossa by the neurosurgery service of the principal military hospital of instruction of Tunis over a period of 16 years between January 2000 and December 2015).

REMINDER ANATOMY

I. General

The posterior cerebral fossa (PCF) is an inextensible osteofibrous cavity located at the posteroinferior part of the base of the skull above the spinal canal[3]. It is the widest and deepest of the three intracranial fossae. Its dimensions, which vary according to breed and individual, are approximately 12 cm wide, 7 cm long and 4 cm high [3].

It extends above the tentorial incision (Paccioni's foramen ovale), through which it communicates with the supratentorial layer, to the foramen magnum at the bottom, where it communicates with the spinal canal.

It is limited [3]: (Figure 1)

- Anteriorly by the dorsal surface of the sella turcica of the sphenoidal bone and by the basilar lamina of the occipital bone;
- Behind and below the broad occipital scale, which is centred by the foramen magnum;
- Above, through the cerebellum tent;
- Laterally on either side, it forms with the lower edge of the rock a the petro-basilar gutter through which the inferior petrosal sinus passes.

Its intracranial base is penetrated by the jugular foramen, the internal auditory meatus and the condylar canal [3-5].

The PCF contains the pathways regulating the level of consciousness and autonomic vital functions, as well as the centres of balance and statics, and the receptors for motor and sensory activity in the head, trunk and extremities. Only the first two pairs of cranial nerves are located entirely outside the PCF; the other ten pairs have a portion within the PCF [4].

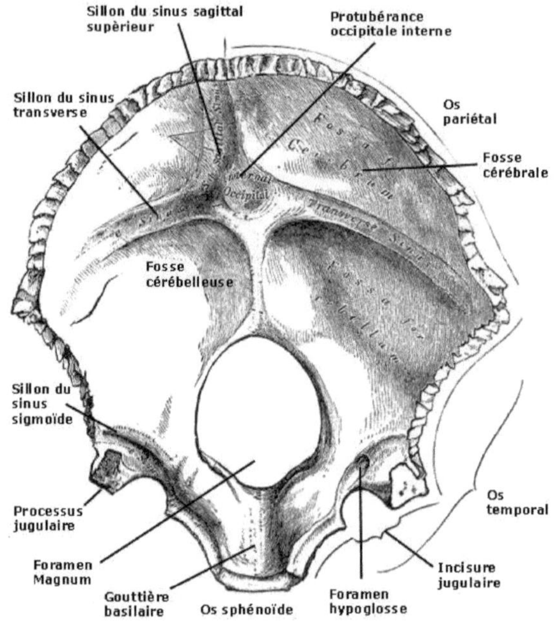

Figure 1: Upper endocranial view showing the bony walls of the PCF.

II. Content of the posterior cerebral fossa

The posterior cerebral fossa contains the brain stem and cerebellum, centred by the 4th ventricle. It also contains the cranial nerves, vessels and meninges.

1. The cerebellum

It is located behind the brainstem (Pons and medulla oblongata) and is separated from the latter in the medial region by the 4ème ventricle [3,5] (Figure 2). It weighs an average of 130 grams in adult men, and measures an average of 10 cm in transverse diameter, 5 to 6 cm in anteroposterior diameter and 6 to 7 cm in height [3].

The cerebellum is connected to the brainstem by three pairs of cerebellar peduncles [3]:

- Superior (brachium conjonctivum) connects the cerebellum to the midbrain;
- Medium connects the cerebellum to the annular protuberance;
- Inferior (restiform and juxtarestiform bodies) connects the cerebellum to the medulla oblongata.

Its surface (cerebellar cortex) is furrowed by numerous roughly transverse furrows separating cerebellar lamellae. The cerebellum consists of two large lateral lobes or cerebellar hemispheres and a medial portion corresponding to the vermis [4,5].

It has three sides:

- The anterior surface covers the roof of the 4th ventricle (V4) at the bulbo-protuberantial level;
- The upper surface is separated from the lower surface of the occipital cortex by the cerebellar tent, which runs obliquely upwards and forwards;
- The inferior or posteroinferior surface is connected to the scale of the occipital bone and its meninges [4-7].

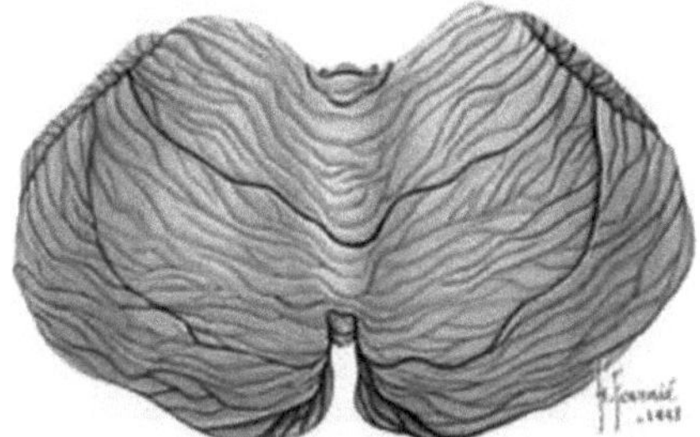

Figure 2: Posterior view of the posterior cerebral fossa showing the cerebellum.

2. The brain stem

It is a transitional structure between the brain and the spinal cord, located in the PCF in front of the cerebellum and covered by the cerebellar tenta;

The brain stem is subdivided into 3 levels from bottom to top [3,4]:
- the medulla oblongata (derived from the myelencephalon) ;
- the annular protuberance, Pons or Varole's bridge (from the metencephalon);
- the mesencephalon or cerebral peduncle.

The brainstem contains all the major ascending and descending pathways (sensory and motor), the nuclei of the cranial nerves and those of the brainstem itself [3]. The ependymal cavity dilates in the brain stem, forming the floor of the 4th ventricle. The reticular substance is a network of neurons intercalated between the preceding structures [3-5]. It supports cortical activity and controls tone.

3. The 4ème ventricle

The 4ème ventricle (V4) is a median cavity between the cerebellum at the back and the brainstem at the front [3,6]. It is connected rostrally via Sylvius' aqueduct to the 3rd ventricle, caudally via Magendie's foramen to the great cistern and laterally via Luschka's foramen to the cisterns of the cerebellopontine angle. The V4 has a roof and a floor [7-10].

3.1. The V4 floor

The floor of V4 is diamond-shaped with a large vertical and median axis. It has a median groove (stem of the Calamus scriptorius) and its short horizontal axis contains the medullary striae. It is then divided into two triangles and an intermediate (junctional) zone [7,9].

- Bottom: the bulbar triangle (posterior surface of the bulb) ;
- Above: the pontic or protuberant triangle ;
- The junction between the 2 triangles.

Its lateral limits are represented by :

- At bulbar level: the two inferior cerebellar peduncles, which connect the bulb to the cerebellum [3].
- At the pontine level: the two superior cerebellar peduncles, which connect the midbrain to the cerebellum [4].
- The junction: the enormous middle cerebellar peduncle, which joins the protuberance to the cerebellum.
- The floor of V4 contains the nuclei of the cranial nerves arranged in columns [3,5].
- In the internal projections: the column of motor cores ;
- In the intermediate depression: columns of vegetative nuclei ;
- In the external projections: columns of sensory and sensory nuclei.

3.2. The roof of the V4

The pontine triangle is formed by a lamina of white matter: the superior medullary veil (Vieussens valve) [3]. The bulbar triangle is limited :

- At the top, the Tarin's valve is a horizontal blade of white substance.
- At the bottom, by the tectorial membrane [5] pierced in the middle by Magendie's foramen and covered by the pie-mother which forms, with the membrane the inferior choroidal web.

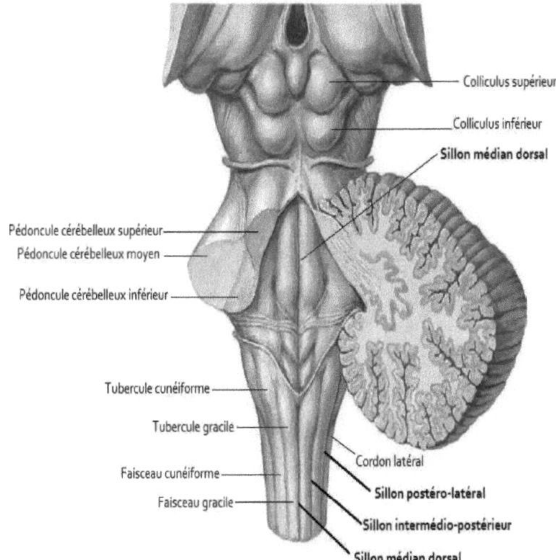

Figure 3: Posterior view showing the bulbar triangle on the floor of V4

4. The cranial nerves

Most of the cranial nerves originate in the brain stem at the anterolateral aspect of the bulb and the Pons, while the last ten cranial nerves cross the arachnoid spaces at the level of the PCF at the cerebellopontine angle to the bony orifices at the base of the skull [5-7].

They fall into three main groups:

► A top group represented by :

▪ The external occulomotor nerve (VI), which arises near the median part of the bulboprotuberan sulcus;

▪ The trigeminal nerve (V), which arises a little higher up on the anterior surface of the protuberance.

► A middle group represented by the acoustic-facial bundle formed by the nerve facial nerve (VII), Wrisberg's intermediate nerve (VIIbis) and the cochleovestibular nerve (VIII), all three of which arise from the outer part of the bulboprotuberantial sulcus.

► A lower group formed by the glosso-pharyngeal (IX), vagus (X) and spinal (XI) nerves, all three of which arise from the posterior collateral sulcus of the bulb.

▪ To these three main groups should be added :

▪ The greater hypoglossal nerve (XII) arises from the lower part of the preolivary sulcus of the bulb;

▪ The common oculomotor nerve (III) and trochlear nerve (IV) emerge from the ventral and dorsal surface of the midbrain respectively [5,7].

5. Meningeal formations

They are formed by cerebrospinal lakes and choroidal formations on the roof of the 4th ventricle.

5.1. The dura mater

It is situated in contact with the bone, forms the venous sinuses by splitting into two and constitutes :

- The cerebellar tent: located between the occipital lobes at the top and the cerebellum at the bottom. It is a fibrous layer stretched over the cranial fossa.

Its medial edge, together with the dorsum sellae, forms the limits of the tentorial incision or foramen of Paccioni. Together with the dorsum sellae, its medial border forms the limits of the tentorial incisure or foramen of Paccioni [4,6].

- The scythe of the cerebellum: located under the tent, it represents an extension of the cerebellum. attached by its posterior edge to the medial occipital crest, and by its posterosuperior edge to the cerebellar tent [4,6].

5.2. The magpie :

It forms the choroid plexus through its membranous extensions, which are made up of two sheets joined by thin trabeculae. These are located in the angle of the cerebellum and the tectorial membrane. They are [4,6].

- the choroid plexuses of the 4th ventricle.

5.3. Tankers

The cisterns are subarachnoid spaces located between the piebrae and the outer membrane of the arachnoid layer, which form several lakes containing cerebrospinal fluid (CSF).

These FCP tanks are represented by :

- The upper cerebellar lake: located between the cerebellar tent and the upper surface of the cerebellum;
- The large cistern: this is an odd numbered cistern which bathes the posteroinferior surface of the cerebellum around the foramen magnum [3,4,6].
- The pre-pontic cistern and the cerebellopontine cisterns: located in front of the anterior surface of the peduncle and cerebellum, against the posterior surface of the cerebellum. du rocher [3, 4,6]

These different arachnoid formations communicate directly with the 4th ventricle via Magendie's and Luschka's holes [6].

III. Vascularisation of the PCF :

1. Arterial vascularisation

The two vertebral arteries give rise to the basilar artery, which in t u r n gives rise to branches intended to vascularise the brain stem and cerebellum [8-10].

1.1. Vertebral artery

It arises from the subclavian artery and has four portions: cervical (v1), vertebral (v2), suboccipital (v3) and intracranial (v4).It enters the skull through the foramen magnum anterior to the greater hypoglossal nerve, and unites with its contralateral counterpart at the level of the pulmonobulbar sulcus to form the basilar artery or basilar trunk [8]. At the level of the PCF, the vertebral artery gives rise to several collaterals:

- spinal arteries (anterior and posterior);
- bulbar branches ;
- the posteroinferior cerebellar artery or PICA, which is the largest branch destined for the choroid plexuses of the 4th ventricle and the cerebellum.

1.2. The basilar trunk

Also known as the basilar artery, it is formed by the union of the two vertebral arteries at the level of the ponto-bulbar sulcus. It roughly follows the basilar sulcus dug into the anterior face of the Pons and has two terminal branches at the level of the ponto-mesencephalic junction: the right and left posterior cerebral arteries [8].

Along the way, it gives rise to the :

- Perforating pontine arteries, irrigating the pons ;
- Anteroinferior cerebellar arteries, supplying the cerebellum and pons ;
- Superior cerebellar arteries, supplying the upper surface of the cerebellum.

Finally, it should be remembered that all these cerebellar terminal branches form a major anastomotic network at the level of the cerebellar convexity, creating a veritable vascular net which surrounds the structures of the posterior fossa [8,9].

2. Venous vascularisation

The venous vascularisation of the PCF is ensured by :

- The bulbar veins, which form a fine pie-merian network draining into the
- the anterior and posterior median veins.
- The cerebellar veins are divided into two groups:

- The vermian or median cerebellar veins, which drain either superiorly into Galen's great vein and the right sinus or inferiorly. in the lower part of the right sinus or in the lateral sinus [10].
- The lateral cerebellar veins drain into two streams: An upper stream that leads to the petrous

sinus and lateral sinus, and a lower stream that leads to the lateral sinus [10].
The veins of the PCF drain into sinuses located in the dura mater [9,10]:

- The right sinus, which runs through the thickness of the cerebellum tent at the level of the insertion of the cerebral scythe [10].
- The superior and inferior petrous sinuses: connect the cavernous sinuses with the transverse sinuses and the internal jugular vein [10].
- The transverse occipital sinus or basilar plexus: runs along the posterior surface of the quadrilateral lamina [10].
- The posterior occipital sinus: runs along the posterior edge of the foramen magnum.
- The torcular or Herophilus press: receives the superior sagittal sinus, the rectus sinus and drains into the transverse and occipital sinuses [9,10].
- The lateral sinus: arises at the level of the torcular, follows the greater circumference of the cerebellar tent to the posterior torn foramen [9,10].

PATIENTS & METHODS

I. Type of study

Our work is a retrospective descriptive study of 25 patients treated at the neurosurgery department of the main military training hospital in Tunis for HED of the FCP, collected over a period of 16 years from January 2000 to December 2015.

II. Population studied

1. Inclusion criteria

We chose to include in the study all cases of CPF HED whose diagnosis was confirmed by brain CT.

2. Exclusion criteria

Not all patients were included in the study:

- Situé en dehors de la période concernée par l'étude
- Dont le diagnostic étiologique reste incertain
- Dont la prise en charge a été faite en dehors du service de neurochirurgie de Tunis Military Hospitalon cerebral CT.

III. Data collection

Epidemiological, clinical and paraclinical data were collected, as well as data relating to the aetiological diagnosis, treatment and outcome.

❖ **Epidemiological data**

We specified age, sex and habits, paying particular attention to alcohol consumption, as well as antecedents such as epilepsy, blood flow disorders, medication use, diabetes and high blood pressure.

❖ **Clinical data**

We noted the time and reason for consultation, the circumstances of the occurrence, the point of cranial impact, the existence of a scalp wound, the notion of initial loss of consciousness and the free interval. We recorded the neurological examination data, in particular the Glasgow score and local signs, the local examination and the general examination. Assessment is based on the Glasgow score (GCS), which evaluates the patient's state of consciousness using three criteria: eye opening, verbal response and best motor response.

Table 1: Glasgow score in adults.

Opening the eyes	Verbal response	Best response motor
4: Spontaneous	5: Oriented	6: Obey the request verbal
3: On request	4: Confused	5 : Pain-oriented
2: To pain	3: Inappropriate	4: Unsuitable avoidance to pain
1 : None	2: Incomprehensible	3: Décortication (Flexion to pain)
	1 : None	2: Decerebration (Extension to pain)
		1 :None

The verbal response is age-appropriate for children.

Table 2: Glasgow score in children.

Opening the eyes	Verbal response	Best response motor
4: Spontaneous	5: Oriented	6: Obey the request verbal
3: On request	4: Words	5: Pain-oriented
2: To pain	3: Sounds	4: Avoidance not adapted to the pain
1 : None	2: Cris	3: Stripping (Flexion to pain)
	1 : None	2: Decerebration (Extension to pain)
		1 :None

❖ **Radiological data**

We have detailed the appearance, location, size, mass effect and other craniocerebral lesions associated with HED in PCF on cerebral CT. We defined the thickness of a HED as the maximum distance between the internal table of the bone and the dura mater. The calculation was based on axial scans. We also noted the existence of associated extra-cranial lesions.

❖ **Therapeutic methods**

We noted the time taken to initiate treatment and the various therapeutic measures undertaken, namely resuscitation and surgical treatment.

❖ **Evolution**

Data on immediate and secondary developments were collected. We assessed functional sequelae using the

Glasgow Outcome Scale (GOS).

This classification is divided into five classes:

- GOS 5 = Good recovery: the patient has resumed a normal life, although he or she may have minor problems.

▪ GOS 4 = Moderate disability: the patient has a disability compatible with a social life; he or she is independent in most activities of daily living.

They can return to work (possibly in a sheltered workshop).

▪ GOS 3 = Severe disability: the patient is conscious but dependent in the activities of daily living; it is impossible to return to work.
▪ GOS 2 = Vegetative state: absence of functioning of the cerebral cortex; it

there is spontaneous breathing; the patient swallows food; he is mute.
▪ GOS 1= Death.
We considered the outcome to be favourable if the GOS was between 5 and 4, and unfavourable if the GOS was less than or equal to 3.

❖ Statistical data capture and analysis

All data were analysed using SPSS software version 21.0. The statistical analysis enabled a descriptive study and an analytical study to be carried out. Qualitative variables were presented as percentages and quantitative variables as averages.

RESULTS

I. Epidemiology

1. Frequency

1.1. Annual incidence

The total number of patients admitted for HED of the posterior cerebral fossa during this period from January 2000 to December 2015 was 25 cases, with an average of 1.56 patients per year.

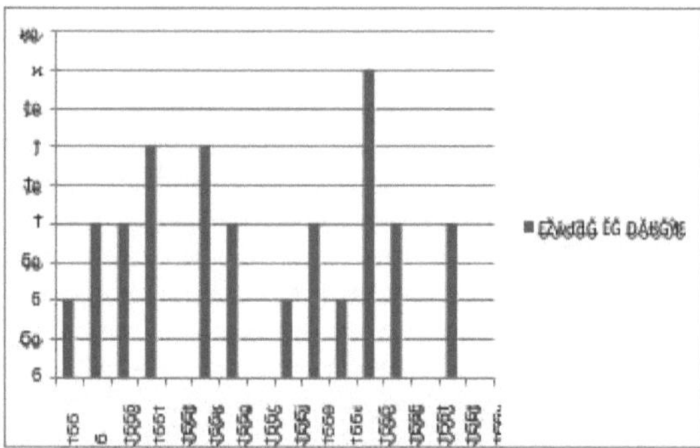

Figure 4: Number of FCP HED cases by year

1.2. Frequency in relation to the total number of extradural haematomas

During the same period, 126 patients were admitted to the Neurosurgery Department for extradural haematoma (EDH), 25 of whom had an extradural haematoma of the posterior cerebral fossa, representing 19.84% of all EDH.

Table 3: Frequency of PCF HEDs as a proportion of total HEDs, by year.

YearNumber of FCP HEDs	Total number of HED	HED of the FCP/HED	
2000	1	10	10%
2001	2	7	28,57%
2002	2	6	33,33%
2003	3	12	25%
2004	0	4	0%
2005	3	8	37,5%
2006	2	9	22,22%
2007	0	7	0%
2008	1	9	11,11%
2009	2	10	20%
2010	1	5	20%
2011	4	15	26,66%
2012	2	8	25%
2013	0	2	0%
2014	2	5	40%
2015	0	9	0%

1.3. Frequency compared with head injuries

During the same period, 619 patients were hospitalised in the Neurosurgery Department for head trauma (CT), 25 of whom had an extradural haematoma of the posterior cerebral fossa, representing 4.03% of all CTs.

Table 4: Frequency of HED in PCF compared with CT, by year.

Year	Number of HEDs in the FCP	Number of TC	FCP/TC HED
2000	1	45	2,22%
2001	2	38	5,26%
2002	2	37	5,40%
2003	3	35	8,57%
2004	0	39	0%
2005	3	35	8.57%
2006	2	36	5,55%
2007	0	40	0%
2008	1	37	2,7%
2009	2	38	5,26%
2010	1	35	2,85%
2011	4	47	8,51%
2012	2	40	5%
2013	0	38	0%
2014	2	42	4,76%
2015	0	37	0%

2. Age

The average age of the population studied was 26.84%, with extremes ranging from 5 to 69 years.Sixteen of our patients (64% of cases) were aged between 16 and 40, while only 05 patients (20% of cases) were over 40. Children accounted for 16% of patients, with 04 cases (any patient aged 15 or under was included in this category).

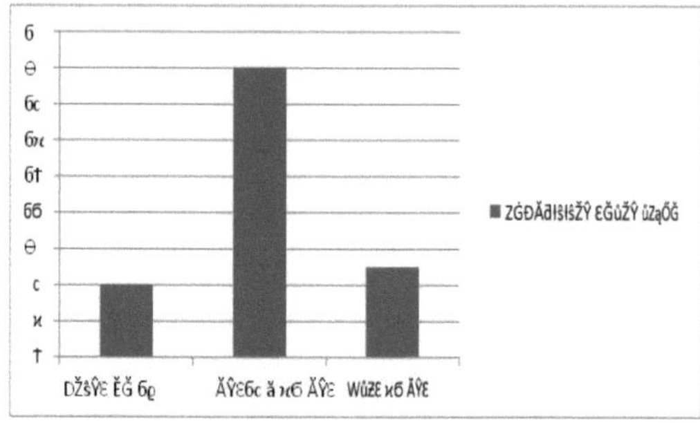

Figure 5: Breakdown of patients by age group.

3. Gender

Our series was predominantly male, with 19 men (76%) and 6 women (24%), giving a sex ratio of 3.16.

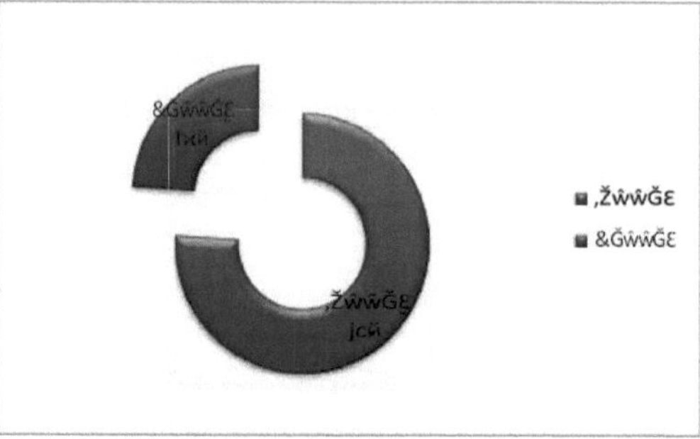

Figure 6: Breakdown of patients by sex.

4. Causes

The aetiologies of trauma are represented by :

- Road accidents: Twelve cases, or 48%.
- Falls: Seven cases, representing 28%.
- Assaults: Six cases, or 24%.

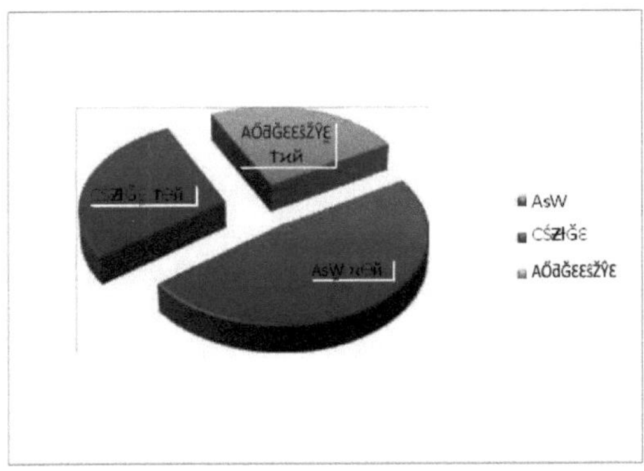

Figure 7: Overall distribution of HED in PCF by aetiology

Taking all ages together, MVAs are the main cause of HED in PCF in our series.

II. Clinic

1. Consultation period

This delay is defined by the time interval between the head injury and the patient's admission to the emergency department. In our series, the average time was 24.08 hours, with extremes ranging from 6 to 80 hours:

- Less than 24 hours in 14 patients (56%).
- One day in 6 patients, i.e. 24%.
- Two days in 3 patients (12%).
- Three days in a single patient, i.e. 4%.
- More than three days in one patient (4%).

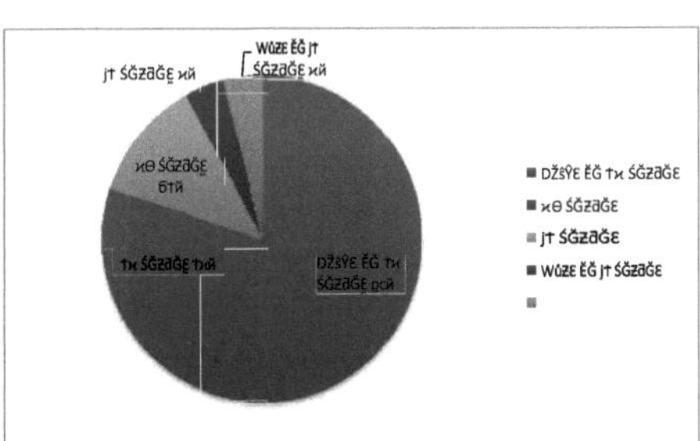

Figure 8: Breakdown of patients by time to consultation

2. Initial loss of consciousness

The notion of an initial loss of consciousness (LOC) was found in 19 patients in the series, i.e. 76%.

3. Free interval

The free interval is defined as the period of time following the cranial trauma which is marked by the absence of any symptomatology. Long considered a classic clinical sign of the three-stage drama of extradural haematoma, it was only found in 14 patients in our series, i.e. 56%.

4. The point of impact

In our series, the mechanism of trauma was direct impact on the nucho-occipital region in 19 patients, i.e. 76% of cases.

5. functional signs

Signs of intracranial hypertension were found in 22 of our patients (88%).

Table 5: Distribution of signs of HTIC in patients

Clinical sign	Number of patients	percentage
Headaches	22	88%
vomiting	20	80%

We have consciousness disorders in 3 of our patients (12%).

6. Clinical examination

6.1. General examination

Haemodynamic status was assessed by measuring pulse and blood pressure, while respiratory status was assessed by respiratory rate. All our patients were haemodynamically and respiratorily stable on admission.

6.2. The state of consciousness

Consciousness was assessed using the Glasgow Coma Score (GCS). Twenty-two of our patients had a GCS of between 13 and 15, 02 patients had a GCS of between 8 and 12 and only one patient had a GCS of less than 7.

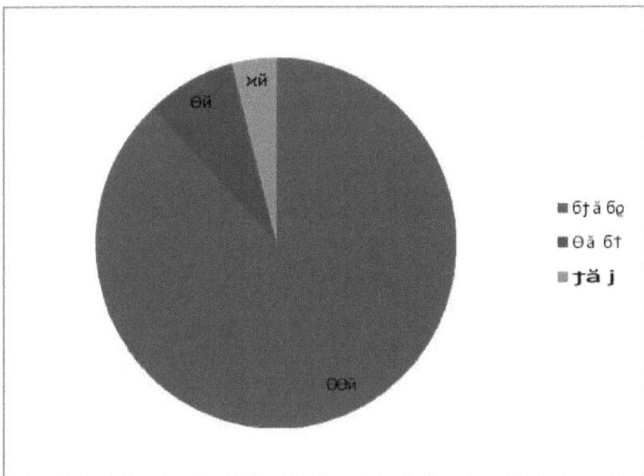

Figure 9: Distribution of patients according to Glasgow score on admission

6.3. Neurological signs

Ten patients had a cerebellar syndrome (40%) and 04 of our patients had a meningeal syndrome (16%).

6.4. Associated lesions

6.4.1 Scalp lesions

Eleven patients had a scalp wound (44%), five had an occipital wound (20%).

6.4.2 Systemic lesions

We reported associated extracranial lesions in 6 patients:

- Four patients had facial and ENT lesions such as facial wounds, epistaxis and otorrhagia.
- Only one patient had abdominal lesions in the form of hepatic contusion.
- One patient had a right rib fracture.
- Two patients had a stable fracture of the thoraco-lumbar hinge.
- Only one patient had a closed fracture of the right upper limb.

III. Radiology

The main complementary examination carried out in all our patients was a cerebral CT scan. This enabled us to determine :

1. The HED headquarters

HED of the PCF was unilateral in all cases, and right-sided in 16 patients.In the case of an occipital fracture, all the HEDs in the PCF were on the same side of the fracture.

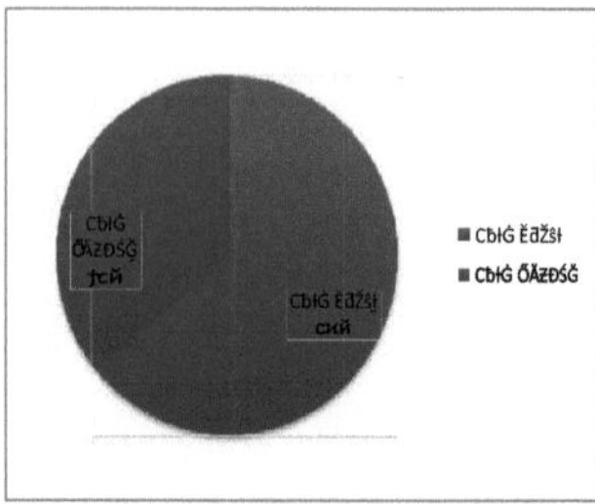

Figure 10: Breakdown of FCP HED by location

2. Aspect of HED

The hyperdense, homogeneous, biconvex lens appearance was found in 20 patients (80%). A heterogeneous hyperdense appearance was found in 4 patients (16%). A hypodense appearance was found in only one patient (4%).

3. Thickness of the HED of the FCP

We divided the HEDs of the FCP into 2 groups according to their thickness:

- the first group: HED thickness less than 10mm (found in 17 patients).
- The second group: HED thickness greater than 10mm (found in 8 patients).

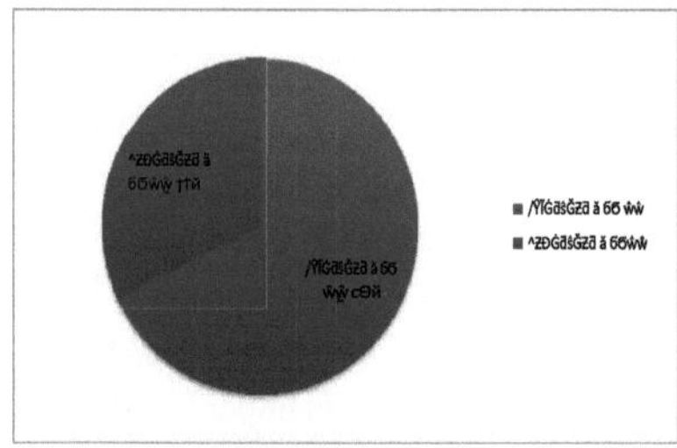

Figure 11: Distribution of HED by thickness

4. The mass effect

In our series, it was found in 8 patients (32%). The mass effect always involved the homolateral cerebellar hemisphere.

5. Skull fracture

We observed a skull fracture in 16 patients (64%).

The fracture site was occipital in 15 patients, representing 93.75% of all fractures and 60% of the overall population.

6. Other cranioencephalic injuries

In 13 patients, we found associated sustentorial parenchymal lesions, such as :

- Sites of haemorrhagic contusions: Six patients.
- Post-traumatic meningeal haemorrhage: Four patients.
- Supra-tentorial HED: Three cases, two of which were occipital and one parietal.
- Pneumencephaly: Three cases.

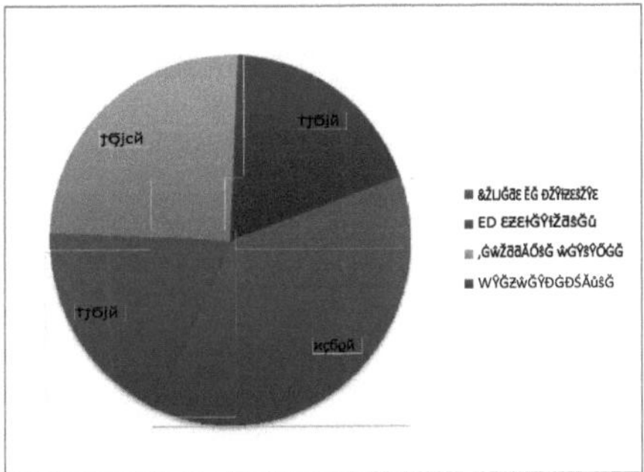

Figure 12: Distribution of different cranioencephalic lesions

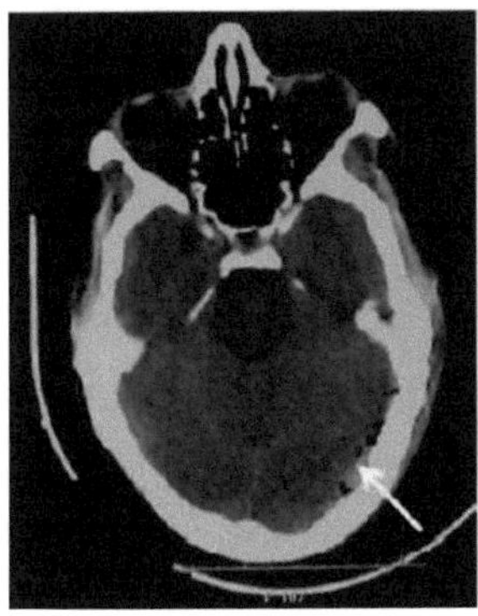

Figure 13: Axial section brain CT scan, parenchymal window showing a lamina of HED of the PCF on the left side associated with bullae of pneumencephaly.

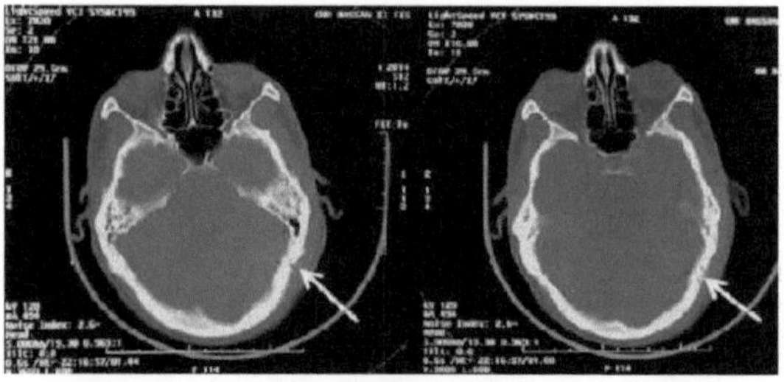

Figure 14: Axial-slice cerebral CT scan, bone windows of the same patient

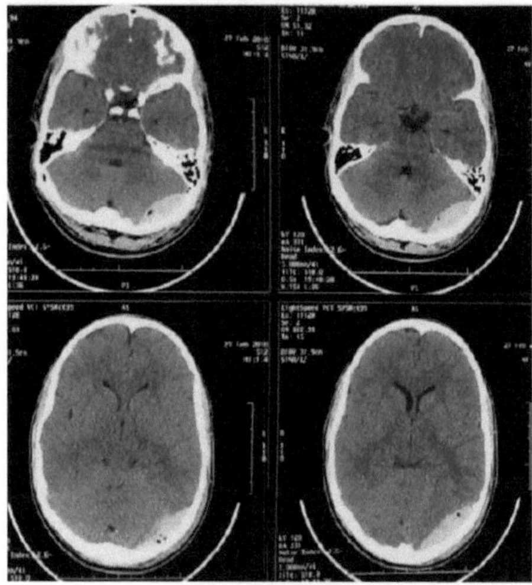

Figure 15: Cerebral CT scan in axial sections, parenchymal windows, showing a frank left HED of the PCF associated with a sustentorial left parieto-occipital HED.

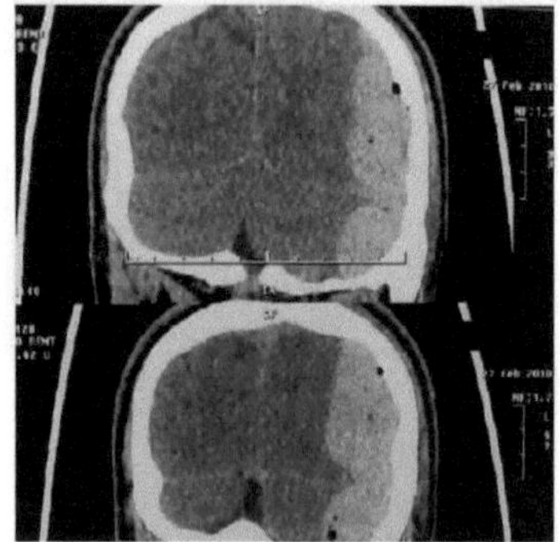

Figure 16: Cerebral CT scan with coronal reconstructions of the same patient as in figure 14, showing a left supratentorial and subtentorial HED associated with extradural pneumocephalus.

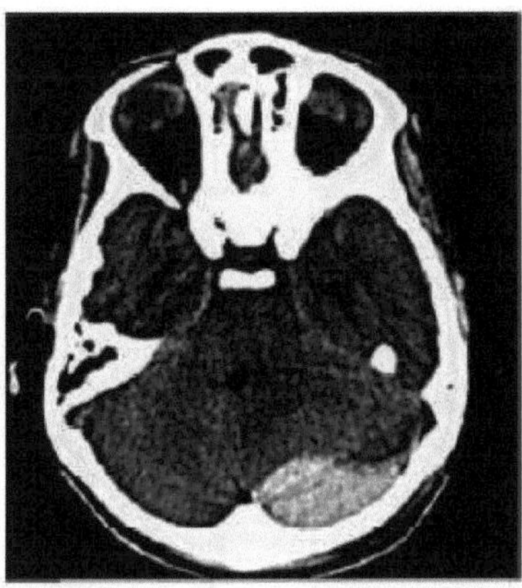

Figure 17: Cerebral CT in axial section, parenchymal window, showing a large compressive right subtentorial HED.

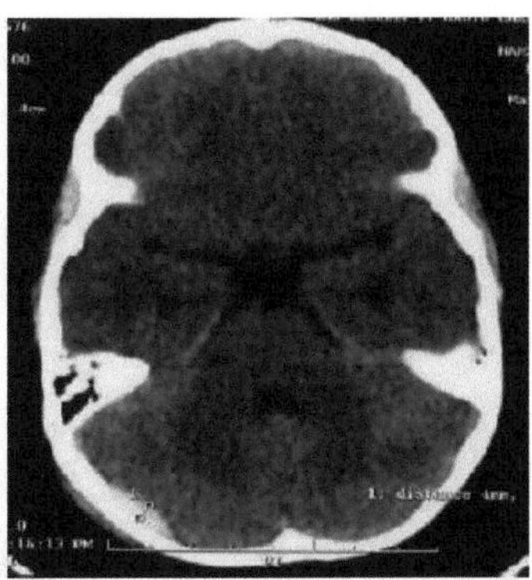

Figure 18: Cerebral CT scan in axial section, parenchymal window, showing a lamina of HED of the PCF on the left.

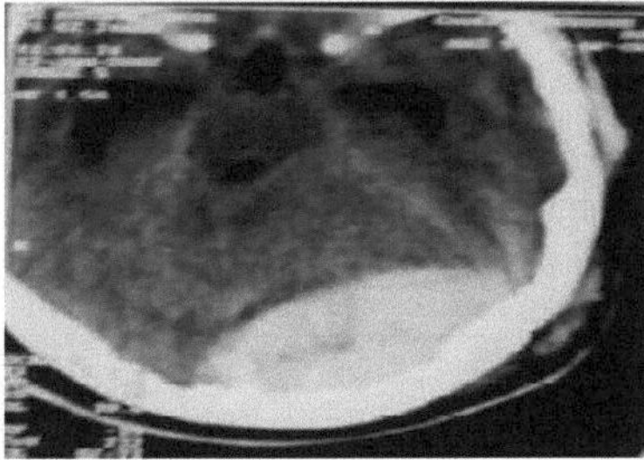

Figure 19: Axial section centred on the PCF of a large compressive left HED.

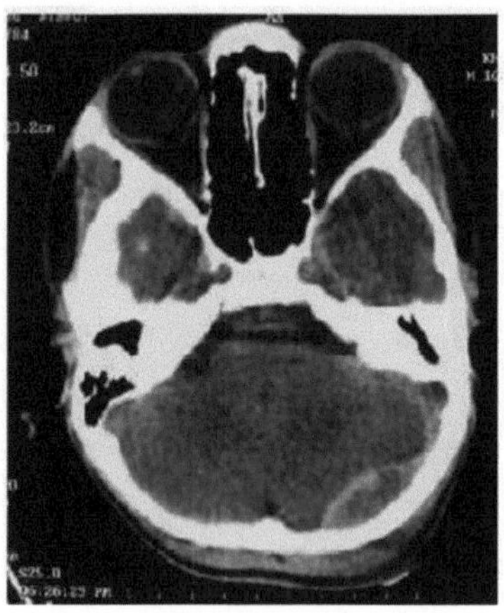

Figure 20: Axial section cerebral CT scan, parenchymal window, showing heterogeneous HED of the left PCF.

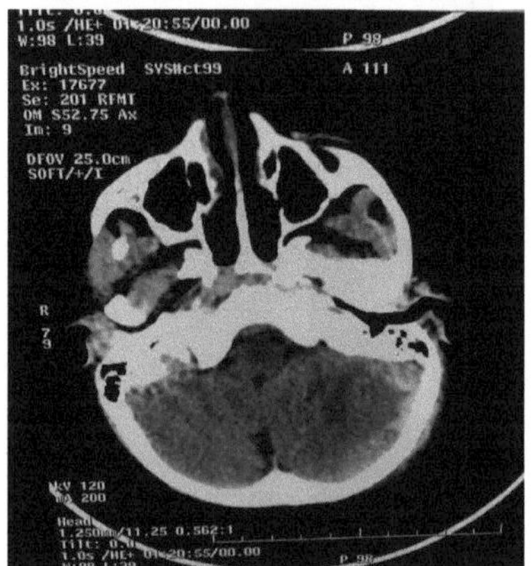

Figure 21: Axial section cerebral CT scan, parenchymal window, showing a heterogeneous HED lamina of the left PCF.

IV. Treatment

1. Therapeutic attitude

HED of the PCF is a neurosurgical emergency. In our series, 8 patients underwent emergency surgery.The indication for surgery was given secondarily in 3 patients, either following a secondary alteration in the state of consciousness or following a follow-up cerebral CT scan showing an increase in the volume of the HED of the FCP. Fourteen patients underwent conservative treatment consisting of symptomatic medical therapy with a good clinical and radiological outcome, with secondary disappearance of the EDH on distant scans.

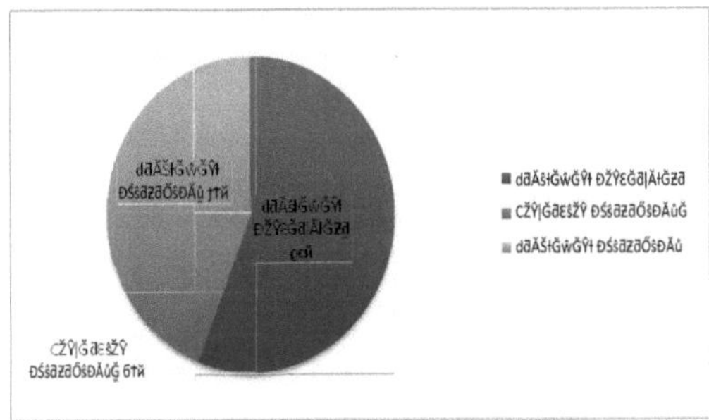

Figure 22: Distribution of patients according to behaviour.

2. Surgical technique

All our patients underwent a sub-occipital bone-through craniectomy combined with evacuation of the haematoma and haemostasis.Only one patient underwent a supratentorial flap at the same time, allowing evacuation of a homolateral sustentorial HED.

3. Origin of bleeding

We were able to determine the origin of the bleeding in 06 of our patients, i.e. 75% of those operated on and 24% of the population as a whole (Table 6, Figure 23).

Table 6: Origin of bleeding

Origin of bleeding	Number of cases
Duremerian sheet	3
Lateral sinus	2
Bone fracture	1
Not found	2

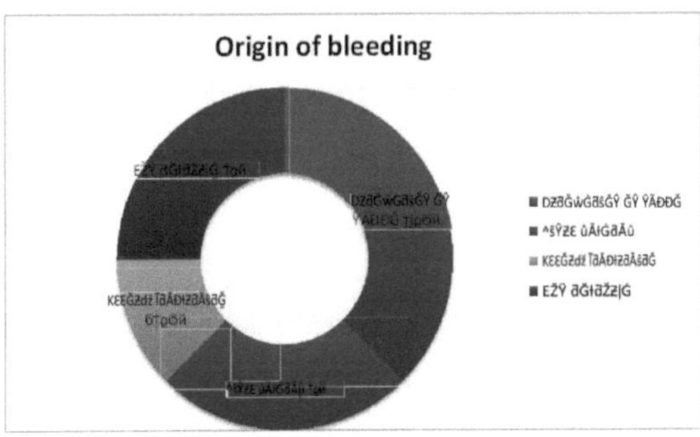

Figure 23: Breakdown of patients by cause of bleeding

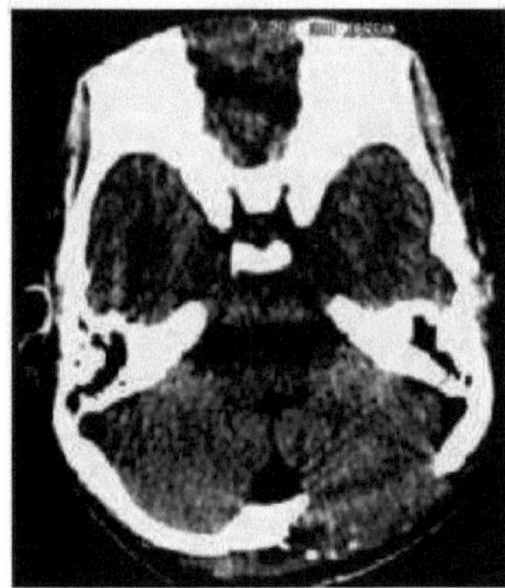

Figure 24: CT scan of the brain of the patient in figure 19, axial section, parenchymal window, showing a right occipital craniectomy with almost complete evacuation of the HED.

V. Course and prognosis

1. Immediate post-operative course

The immediate post-operative course was straightforward in all our patients.

2. Mortality

There were no deaths in our series.

3. Functional prognosis

The outcome was favourable in 23 patients (Table 7).

Table 7: Breakdown of patients by functional prognosis

Evolution	GOS	Number of patients	Percentage
Favourable	5 and 4	23	92%
Unfavourable	3 and 2	2	8%

DISCUSSION

I. Epidemiology

1. Frequency

HED of the PCF is a rare but not exceptional lesion. At the beginning of the twentieth century, it was generally discovered during autopsies, which made it difficult to establish the exact frequency of this lesion.In recent years, the number of PCF HEDs diagnosed has risen sharply thanks to the development of neuroradiological investigations, particularly CT. In 1990, Thierry et al [11] reported 20 cases of HED of the FCP treated in 10 years, i.e. approximately 6.5% of all HED. In 1996, Costa Clara et al[12] described in their series 3 cases of HED of the PCF among 31 HED, i.e. 9.7%, and among 2372 head injuries, i.e. 1.3%. In 2001, A. Kabre et al [13] reported 130 cases of supratentorial and subtentorial HED, of which 20 cases were located in the PCF, i.e. 14.3% of cases. In 2007, Toshiaki Hayashi et al[14] reported 21 HED of the PCF out of a total of 251 HED, estimating that this entity represented 8.4% of all HED. In 2008, Roka YB et al [15] described 43 FCP HED in a series of 432 HED, estimating its frequency at around 10% of cases. Bogdan Asanin [16] estimated that FCP HED represented 7.9% of all HED and 0.11% of all TC. In 2014 the Moroccan series by Meknassi [18]described 29 cases of FCP HED among 425 HED or 6.8% of cases and among 7221 TC or 0.97%.Our study was retrospective and involved 25 cases of FCP HED among 126 HED and 619 TC managed, collated over a period of 16 years, from January 2000 to December 2015 (Table 8, Table 9).

Table 8: Number of CPF HEDs compared with the total number of HEDs according to the authors.

Author	Year	Total number of FCP HED cases	Percentage of all HEDs
Thierry et al [11]	1990	10	6,5%
Costa Clara and	1996	3	9,7%
al[12]			
A.Kabre et al	2001	20	14,3%
[13]			
Toshiaki Hayashi	2007	21	8,4%
et al [14]			
Roka YB et al	2008	43	10%
[15]			
Bogdan Asanin	2009	18	7,9%
[16]			
Meknassi [18]	2014	29	6,8%
Our series	2015	25	19,84%

Table 9: Number of FCP HEDs in relation to the total number of CTs according to the authors.

Author	Year	Percentage of FCP HED compared to all CT
Cuirea et al[17]	1993	0,13%
Costa Clara et al[12]	1996	1,3%
Roka YB et al[15]	2008	0,4%
Bogdan Asanin[16]	2009	0,11%
Meknassi[18]	2014	0,37%
Our series	2015	4,03%

HED appears to be the most common post-traumatic lesion of the PCF in the literature. The series by Brown [1] of 21 observations reported 8 HED, 4 HSD, 7 subdural hygromas and 2 intracerebellar haematomas with a percentage ofHED of the PCF of 38.09%. The series by Dirim et al [19] of 49 cases found 7 HED, i.e. 14.2%.

2. Age

The average age of the population studied was 26.84%, with extremes ranging from 5 to 69 years. This result is in line with the majority of series in the literature, which conclude that HED of the PCF is a pathology of the young adult par excellence (table 10).

Table 10: Average age according to authors.

Author	Year	Average age
A.Kabre et al [13]	2001	27 years old
Edson Bor Sen-Shu et al [21]	2004	18.3 years
Toshiaki Hayashi et al[14]	2007	25.6 years
Aykut Karasu et al[20].	2008	16.4 years old
Bogdan Asanin[16]	2009	21.2 years old
Jae-won-jang et al [22]	2011	23.1 years old
Meknassi[18]	2014	25.4 years old
Our series	2015	26.84 years old

3. Gender

Our series was predominantly male, with 19 men (76%) and 6 women (24%), i.e. a sex ratio of 3.16. This male predominance has also been found in most studies of HED in PCF.

Table 11: Breakdown of patients by sex for the different authors.

Author	Year	Total number of cases	Men	women	Sex ratio
Thierry et al	1990	20	16	04	4
[11]					
Ersalin [27]	1993	9	05	04	1,25
Costa Clara		1996	03	01	3
A. Kabre et al [13]	2001	20	18	02	9
Edson Bor	2004	43	33	10	3,3
Sen-Shu et al					
[21]					
Toshiaki	2007	21	14	07	Ŧ
Hayashi and					
al[14]					
Aykut Karasu	2008	65	47	18	2,61
et al[20]					
Bogdan	2009	18	14	04	3,5
Asanin [16]					
Meknassi[18]	2014	29	23	06	3,83
Our series	2015	25	19	6	3,16

4. auses

Aetiology is a contingent that can be acted upon to prevent head injuries and reduce their severity.In our study, the aetiologies were dominated by MVAs, which accounted for 48%, followed by falls (28%) and assaults (24%). Edson Bor-Seng-Shu [21] in 2004 found that the most frequent aetiology was falls in 26 patients (60%), followed by stroke in 17 patients. Toshiaki Hayashi et al [14] in 2007 found that the most common aetiology was stroke in 14 patients (66%), followed by falls in 6 patients (28%) and assault in one patient (4.76%). Aykut Karasu et al [20], in a study of 65 cases in 2008, found that the most common aetiology of HED was stroke in 35 cases (53%), followed by falls in 30 patients.Thus, we found that MVAs provided the largest contingent in the various series in the literature. We also found that in children, the proportion is reversed and falls are the main cause of HED in CPF [21,28,29]. In our series, falls accounted for 75% of the causes of PCF in patients under 15 years of age, exceeding strokes, which represent 25% of the population.

II. Anatomopathology

Typically, post-traumatic HED is temporoparietal in location and is often due to rupture of the middle meningeal artery and/or its branches.HED of the PCF is rarer and more serious [39]. This injury is most often the result of direct trauma to the cervico-occipital region and is usually accompanied by a fracture of the bone opposite [39,40]. The origin of the bleeding may be the lateral sinus in its transverse portion, the Herophilus or torcular pressor or the posterior meningeal artery, which may be sheared or perforated during the trauma [40].

1. Soft tissue injuries

They are virtually constant at the point of impact of the trauma. They vary from a simple bruise that does not break the skin to a wide variety of skin wounds. Subcutaneous bruising and haematomas are not uncommon [40-42].

2. Bone and dural lesions

The bone is the second line of defence against trauma, but its resistance is not uniform. The occipital and temporal scales and the frontal sinus are areas of weakness. As a result, direct impact can cause linear or comminuted fractures, or even embarrure. This depends on the nature of the damaging agent and the energy developed by the trauma [41]. Certain bone injuries can lead to underlying dural lesions: embarrures or comminuted fractures.

3. Associated endocranial lesions

They are produced at the time of the trauma or in its aftermath, and may be diffuse or multiple and distant, suggesting counter-blow lesions. These lesions are partly responsible for the frequent complexity of the initial picture and the worsening prognosis. Cerebral CT can be used to assess them [23-26].

III. Pathophysiology

1. Etiopathogenesis

HED of the PCF is an injury that most often results from direct trauma to the cervico-occipital region. It is usually accompanied by ICP and a skull fracture crossing the lateral sinus, transverse sinus, torcular or posterior meningeal artery, which may be sheared or perforated during the trauma. The point of impact may also be minimal, causing only a simple occipital swelling, with no ICP and no fracture[40]. During trauma, the dura mater may detach from the bone and cause haemorrhage into the extradural space thus created, especially when the fracture line crosses the path of a meningeal vessel. However, in some cases the origin of the bleeding is not found [40].

2. Factors influencing the expansion of HED

According to the literature, certain factors other than the origin of the bleed may play an important role in the expansion of the haematoma. The most important of these are the reduction of intracranial hypertension and cerebral oedema by anti-oedematous treatment (the oedema and ICCH are thought to act as buffers for the source of the haemorrhage) [43,44,52]. The presence of a change in haemodynamic status (in favour of hypertension) or the existence of haemostasis disorders with reduced coagulability. Finally, there is the natural tendency for a haematoma to increase in volume [43].

3. Mechanisms for absorbing HED

Authors have done very little to elucidate these mechanisms. A basic reference is represented by the work of Pang D et al [44], who observed that the mechanisms of HED resorption are comparable to those of subdural haematoma. In agreement with Linderberg [44], he suggested that resorption took place through the "fibrovascular neo-membrane" which covers the dural surface of chronic HED. This capsule, histologically similar to the membrane of the chronic subdural haematoma, has been found in a good number of HEDs reported in the literature. Tuncer et al [45] hypothesised that another mechanism of resorption was the development of arteriovenous shunts in the epidural space during haemorrhage, which would play an important role in the resorption of HED. Kaufman [46] described another potential mode of resorption. In his opinion, it could be secondary to the infiltration of blood through the fracture line opposite the HED. Aoki [47] confirmed this hypothesis by observing that the volume of HEDs decreased simultaneously with the increase in the volume of epicranial haematomas in these patients with a fracture line separating the two collections.

IV. Clinic

1. Consultation period

In our series, the average consultation time was 24.08 hours, with extremes ranging from 6 to 80 hours, which is in line with most results in the literature (Table 12).

Table 12: Consultation times according to authors.

Author	Year	Consultation period in hours
Hayashi et al [14]	2007	22
Karasu et al [20]	2008	26,58
Meknassi [18]	2014	20,89
Our series	2015	24,08

2. The free interval

The notion of a free interval was found in 14 patients (56%).

Table 13: Percentage of free interval recovered according to authors.

Author	Year	Percentage
Thierry et al [11]	1990	15%
A.Kabre et al [13]	2001	40%
Cataltepe O [57]	2003	85%
Nagi et al [49]	2007	25%
Malik et al [60]	2007	36%
Meknassi [18]	2014	51,7%
Our series	2015	56%

Since it was first described by J.L.PETIT in 1750, the notion of free interval has become an essential element in the evaluation of head injuries. It can vary from a few hours to a few days or even a few months in chronic forms [25,26,,28,29,33,34].the free interval is is defined as the period of lucidity following the occurrence of the cranial trauma. This notion must be sought by meticulous questioning of the patient or his entourage. However, it is sometimes difficult to ascertain this notion, as patients may be admitted in a coma, and these patients are often unaccompanied, which partly explains the variability of results between different series in the literature. Currently, authors tend to distinguish between "lucid interval" (secondary appearance of consciousness disorders) and "free interval" (secondary appearance of neurological signs, without major consciousness disorders). This allows a more detailed semiological analysis and early diagnostic guidance.

3. The point of impact

The mechanism of trauma was direct impact to the cervico-occipital region in 19 patients (76%).Trauma to the cervico-occipital region reported with such frequency that some authors have made it a key factor in orienting the diagnosis.

Table 14: Percentage of the point of impact according to the authors.

Author	Year	frequency of trauma to the region cervico-occipital
Belotti et al [31]	1987	72%
Thierry et al [11]	1990	85%
A.Kabre et al [13]	2001	95%
Toshiaki Hayashi et al [14]	2007	66%
Bogdan Asanin [16]	2009	90%
Our series	2015	76%

4. Functional signs

Signs of intracranial hypertension were found in 22 of our patients, i.e. 88% of cases, with headaches in 88% of cases and vomiting in 80%. After reviewing the literature, we noted that signs of ICCH are frequent in extradural haematomas of the posterior cerebral fossa, which is consistent with the results found in our study.

Table 15: Percentage of signs of HTIC according to the authors.

Author	Year	Percentage of signs HTIC
Edson Bor-Seng-shu et al [21]	2004	85,8%
Aykut Karasu et al[20].	2008	76%
Roka YB et al [15]	2008	67,4%
Altay Sencer et al [28]	2012	57,5%
Meknassi [18]	2014	79,3%
Our series	2015	88%

Intracranial Hypertension Syndrome (ICHS) is defined as a set of symptoms related to increased pressure inside the cranium.

It is manifested by :

- Headaches.
- Vomiting: this is more infrequent than headaches and occurs in a flurry, relieving the headache.
- Visual problems, often delayed.

5. Clinical examination :

5.1. General review :

The search for an extra-cranial lesion should be systematic in all skull trauma patients. In fact, polytrauma with neurotrauma makes initial management more complex. On the one hand, the initial clinical examination is often of little help, due to consciousness disorders (occultation effect). This means that extracranial lesions must be systematically sought, as they will condition the management[35,37]. On the other hand, hypoxaemia, linked to a thoraco-pulmonary lesion, whether or not associated with hypotension due to hypovolaemia (summation and amplification effect), obviously aggravates a cranial trauma and can also create a neurological picture which disappears or becomes minor once these two vital constants have been restored [45,47]. A distinction is therefore made between unstable patients who have not been stabilised by resuscitation and stable patients, making it possible to prioritise the management strategy [45,47,53].

5.2. State of consciousness

Assessing and monitoring consciousness is the cornerstone of the management of any cranial trauma.Assessment is based on the Glasgow score (GCS), which evaluates the patient's state of consciousness using three criteria: eye opening, verbal response and best motor response. The GCS is obtained by adding the values of the three criteria, giving an overall score of between 3 and 15. Developed by Teasdale and Jennet in 1974, it is recognised as a reliable tool for assessing the state of consciousness following head trauma and as a criterion for predicting mortality [53-59]. In recent French studies, 30% to 50% of doctors questioned used the GCS inappropriately [53]. The rules to be respected when calculating the GCS are :

- The use of validated nociceptive stimulation methods such as pressure on the supraorbital area or pressure on the nail bed with a pen.
- When the opening of the eyes cannot be assessed in the event of ecchymosis or eyelid oedema. A global GCS cannot be calculated. Scoring is therefore based on responses that can still be assessed.
- In the event of asymmetric responses, the best response is taken into account obtained for each GCS criterion.
- The reference score is obtained after correction for any arterial hypotension and/or hypoxia.
- The GCS should not be reduced to an overall figure, but should describe the three components of the score in figures.
- The GCS cannot be assessed in the context of intoxication or the use of medication that alters the state of consciousness.

Table 16: Distribution of GCS on admission according to authors.

Author	Year	GCS between 13 and 15	GCS between 8 and 12	GCS between 3 and 7
Toshiaki Hayashi et al	2007	18 (85,7%)	1 (4,76%)	2 (9,52%)
[14]				
Aykut Karasu	2008	53 (81%)	) 7 (10%)	5 (8%)
et al[20]				
Roka YB et al	2008	29 (67%)	12 (28%)	2 (5%)
[15]				
Bogdan	2009	(16) 8 (44%)	7 (39%)	3 (19%)
Asanin [16]				
Jae-won-jang et al	2011	22 (64,7%)	6 (17,6%)	6 (17,6%)
[22]				
Meknassi	2014	24 (82,75%)	4 (13,8%)	1 (3,44%)
[18]				
Our series	2015	22 (88%)	2 (8%)	1 (4%)

One criticism of the GCS has been its failure to incorporate brainstem reflexes. A number of authors have disagreed with Teasdale and Jennett that spontaneous eye opening is sufficiently indicative of the activity of brainstem arousal systems and have developed other coma scales that include brainstem responses. These resulting scales have generally been more complex than the GCS [53-57].

The Glasgow-Liege Scale was invented in 1982 by Jacques D. Born and his colleagues, with the aim of improving the GCS, took the Glasgow Scale and added a specific section corresponding to the evaluation of brainstem reflexes, demonstrating that the predictive effectiveness of brainstem reflexes was better than that of motor response. The use of these two parameters in a single scale, the Glasgow-Liège Scale, improves the accuracy of prognosis for patients with severe head injury. The GLS extends the sensitivity of the GCS in phases of deep coma, but is no more sensitive for assessing patients in a vegetative state or in a state of minimal consciousness[57-60].

Brain stem reflexes :

▪ The fronto-orbicular reflex: percussion of the frontal supraorbital region at the level of the glabella physiologically causes bilateral contraction of the orbicularis muscles. This reflex is abolished from stage III (mesodiencephalic) coma onwards.

▪ The vertical oculocephalic reflex: this is sought after ensuring the integrity of the cervical spine, by making sudden movements of the head

of flexion-extension. The normal response is a combined deviation of the eyes on the opposite side to the movements. This is known as the doll's eyes phenomenon. In the case of rosto-caudal deterioration, it disappears in stage III of meso-diencephalic coma.

▪ The photo-motor reflex (PMR): abolished in the event of injury

mesencephalic (stage IV).

▪ The horizontal oculocephalic reflex: a sudden rotation of the head to one side and then the other normally causes a conjugated deviation.

the eyes on the opposite side. The eyes passively follow the movements of the head from the protuberant level V of the coma.

▪ The oculo-cardiac reflex: this corresponds to the slowing down of the heart rate. by the pressure of the eyeballs. This reflex only disappears in the event of bulbar damage [53,57,60].

5.3. Local neurological signs

Regardless of how alert the patient is, neurological signs of localisation must be systematically sought. These signs are often rare and misleading.Edson Bor-Seng-Shu et al [21] observed diplopia in 16.3% of his patients. Aykut Karasu et al [20] noted a cerebellar syndrome in 30% of patients and anisocoria in 7%. Altay Sencer et al [28] found a cerebellar syndrome in 27.5% of cases. Meknassi [18] found a cerebellar syndrome in 34.5% of patients. Roka YB et al [15] found VI paralysis in 2.3% of patients and VII involvement in 2.3%. In our series, we found a cerebellar syndrome in 10 patients (40%), which is in line with the results of the literature.

5.4. Associated lesions

An examination of the scalp should be carried out systematically in all head trauma patients:

- The existence of a scalp wound, which may be responsible for significant blood loss, leading to haemorrhagic shock, especially in children.
- The existence of a loss of scalp substance which may require a lining procedure.
- The existence of a scalp haematoma and an assessment of its size.
- The existence of a deformity of the arch, which points to a fracture with embrasure.
- Cerebral death in the context of a craniocerebral wound, the prognosis of which can be critical. [16, 20,57].

In our series, 11 patients had a scalp wound (44%), five of whom had an occipital wound (20%).

V. Radiology

1. Computed tomography (CT) of the brain

1.1. Contribution of CT

All our patients underwent cerebral CT without injection of contrast medium. CT is an exploratory technique which was presented at the annual meeting of the British Institute of Radiology by Hounsfield in 1972 [68].Cerebral CT will be performed without injection of contrast medium, using 5 to 9 mm thick contiguous slices extending from the foramen magnum to the vertex. It enables a complete and accurate assessment of the lesions to be made urgently, and the therapeutic strategy to be guided. It can also be used to monitor patients during treatment and for follow-up after treatment has been completed [61]. Currently, cerebral CT without contrast injection represents the Gold Standard for radiological exploration in the acute phase in head trauma patients according to the 2016 recommendations of the American College of Radiology [61]. Cerebral CT can be performed quickly and easily in the context of a traumatic emergency, unlike MRI, which takes longer and is difficult to perform in an intubated and ventilated patient. In addition, the possible existence of intracranial ferromagnetic metallic foreign bodies in a recent trauma patient constitutes a risk of severe complications. In the case of HED of the PCF, cerebral CT can unambiguously demonstrate the haematoma, determine its location, appearance, thickness and the existence of a mass effect [61,63].Bone lesions in the vault and base of the skull can also be studied in the bone window and on different sections [63]. Finally, a CT scan may be used to look for associated intracranial lesions. The advent of cerebral CT was a major turning point in the management of CT and contributed significantly to the improvement in prognosis [61,63].

1.2. The HED headquarters

In our series, the HED of the PCF was unilateral in all patients, and on the right side in 16 patients (64%). In the case of occipital fractures, all PCF HEDs were on the same side of the fracture. In 2004, Edson Bor-Seng-Shu et al [21] found that among 43 PCF HEDs, 13 patients (30.23%) had a right-sided haematoma, 17 patients (39.53%) had a left-sided haematoma and in the remaining 13 patients (30.23%), the haematoma was bilateral.In the series by Aykut Karasu et al published in 2008 [20] and involving 65 patients, he found that 23 HED of the PCF were located on the right (35.38%), 35 were on the left (53.84%) and in 7 patients the HED of the PCF was bilateral (10.76%). In the series by Roka YB et al in 2008 [15]. All HED in PCF were unilateral with 81% located on the right.

1.3. Aspect of HED

The appearance of a spontaneously hyperdense, biconvex, well-limited, extra-axial effusion located between the internal table of the bone and the parenchyma, which stops at the sutures and forms an obtuse angle with the bone, is pathognomonic of HED [61]. However, the homogeneity of this appearance varies according to the time between the trauma and the CT scan.

Aykut Karasu et al [20] classified HEDs according to appearance into 3 categories:

- Acute HED with hyperdense CT in 59 patients (90%).
- Subacute HED with isodense brain parenchyma in 4 patients (6%).
- Chronic HED with a heterogeneous hypodense appearance in 2 patients (3%).

In our series, the hyperdense, homogeneous, biconvex lens appearance was found in 20 patients (80%). The heterogeneous hyperdense appearance was found in 4 patients (16%) and the hypodense appearance was found in only one patient (4%).

1.4. The mass effect

Altay Sencer et al [28] found a mass effect in 75% of patients. In our series, it was found in 08 of our patients, i.e. 32% of cases. The mass effect always concerned the homolateral cerebellar hemisphere.

1.5. Skull fracture

A. Kabre et al [13], in a study of 20 cases of HED in PCF, found 17 occipital fractures, i.e. 85%; Toshiaki Hayashi et al [14] found 20 occipital fractures on cerebral CT in a study of 21 patients, i.e. 95.23%. Altay Sencer et al [28] found 35 occipital fractures on cerebral CT, representing 87.5% of patients. We observed a skull fracture in 16 of our patients (64%).
The fracture site was occipital in 15 patients, representing 93.75% of all fractures and 60% of the overall population.

1.6. Other cranioencephalic injuries

We found associated sustentorial parenchymal lesions in 13 of our patients. Focal areas of haemorrhagic contusions in 6 patients, post-traumatic meningeal haemorrhage in 4 patients, pneumencephaly in 3 patients and sustentorial HED in 3 patients, two of which were occipital and one parietal.After reviewing the literature, we noted that foci of cerebral haemorrhagic contusions are the brain lesions most consistently found in association with HED in PCF. Edson Bor-Seng-shu et al [21] analysed 43 HED in PCF and found the following associated cerebral lesions: Contusion foci in 14 patients, cerebral oedema in 5 patients, supratentorial HED in 4 patients, acute subdural haematoma in 3 patients and meningeal haemorrhage in 2 patients.Toshiaki Hayashi et al [14] noted foci of contusion in 10 cases, meningeal haemorrhage in 5 cases and acute subdural haematoma in 3 patients. Aykut Karasu et al reported on 65 PCF HEDs with foci of contusion in 15 cases, supratentorial HED in 07 cases, hydrocephalus in 5 cases, pneumencephalus in 4 cases, cerebral oedema in 2 cases, meningeal haemorrhage in one case and acute subdural haematoma in one case. Finally, Roka YB et al [15] found hydrocephalus in 9 cases, foci of contusions in 08 cases and supratentorial HED in 2 cases. The results of our study concerning associated intraparenchymal lesions are in line with those found in the literature.

1.7. Time taken for CT scan

The time taken to perform a CT scan is defined as the time interval between the occurrence of the trauma and the first CT scan performed on the patient. According to Benmoussa et al [41], this delay is the only indisputable factor in the possible growth ofa HED. He reported that the shorter the delay, the greater the risk of the haematoma increasing in volume, demonstrating that HED is an expansive lesion as a function of time [71]. This contradicts the theory of Ford and Mc Lauron, who asserted that HED reaches its maximum formation in a few minutes [72].Servadei et al [73] also confirmed that HEDs and intracranial haemorrhages are the lesions most likely to worsen secondarily, and found that in comatose patients, if the CT scan was performed before the 3rd hour, it should be repeated within the following 12 hours. In 1992, Poon WS et al [74] confirmed this theory by finding a delayed onset ofHED in 30% of patients who had a CT scan less than one hour after the trauma. Consequently, a normal brain CT scan does not definitively rule out delayed-onset HED, especially when it is performed too early. Clinical monitoring should take this into account, especially in patients with skull fractures [61, 72,74].

Fankhauser et al [75] determined precise criteria for performing a follow-up cerebral CT scan:

- After 48 to 72 hours, a CT scan showed a non-surgical haematoma associated with a fracture.
- In the event of secondary alteration of the state of consciousness or in the event of the appearance of signs of HTIC or signs of localisations.
- If there is no clinical improvement or if the monitored intracranial pressure remains high after evacuation of an intracranial haematoma.
- Systematically after 12 to 24 hours in all head trauma patients under sedation and respiratory

assistance, given the impossibility of assessing the state of consciousness. consciousness and the various clinical signs.

2. Other complementary examinations

2.1. Standard skull X-ray

Standard films can be used to detect a linear or stellate fracture of the vault, disjunction of the sutures, a foreign body or significant pneumencephalus [62].

It should be emphasised that arch lesions are not an indicator of intracranial lesions. In fact, 90% of patients with fractures have no underlying intracranial lesions and 50% of patients with intracranial lesions have no bone lesions [62].

The standard X-ray consists of 4 views:
- Face.
- 2 profiles: right and left.
- Occiput incision on Worms-Breton plate: this is of considerable importance, as it provides a much better view of the PCF as far as the foramen magnum. In the case of HED of the PCF, the skull fracture most often crosses the path of the lateral sinus or the torcular [62]. However, standard radiography may omit the fracture in up to 15% of cases. [63, 64].

Since the advent of CT, the indications for standard radiography have been significantly reduced [65]. In addition to the false security offered by the absence of a skull fracture, it has been widely demonstrated that intracranial lesions can occur despite the absence of any bone lesion [66]. We therefore concluded that in a hospital with a CT scanner, standard skull X-rays have no place in the management of head trauma.

2.2. Cerebral angiography

When it comes to HED, we cannot do justice without mentioning the fundamental role played by cerebral angiography for over 50 years. It was once considered the gold standard in trauma neuroimaging. It has been largely overtaken by CT, which is quicker and easier to perform.At present, diagnostic cerebral angiography no longer has a place in the hierarchy of examinations requested in the acute phase of a head injury [76]. The typical clinical appearance is that of an avascular biconvex lens, corresponding to the detachment of the cortical vessels. Sometimes a puddle of contrast medium can be seen in the wound of the meningeal artery (Lindgren's sign). An associated circulatory slowdown indicates parenchymal lesions with a poor prognosis [76].

2.3. Magnetic resonance imaging (MRI)

CT may miss a HED at the level of the clivus [77]. This location at the level of the PCF can be confirmed by MRI, which is not affected by cranial bone artefacts.Kurosu et al [77] reported a case of HED of the clivus diagnosed by MRI in an 11-year-old patient who had been involved in a road traffic accident (RTA) with ICP. CT revealed a subarachnoid haemorrhage with no other associated abnormalities. The course was marked by a secondary alteration in consciousness associated with tetraparesis. Another cerebral CT scan was performed, showing no intracranial haematoma, but a high density in the clivus, and a cerebro-spinal MRI was ordered, showing no HED in the small clivus. Conservative treatment was chosen with a good outcome.Orisson et al [78] compared the contribution of CT and MRI in the management of CT in 107 observations. He showed that MRI was more sensitive than CT in detecting contusions, subdural and extradural haematomas, while CT was more sensitive in detecting fractures. The sensitivity of these two examinations was statistically equivalent in the detection of superficial soft tissue lesions. The sensitivity of MRI in detecting abnormalities during acute CT was 94.4%, compared with 63.4% for CT [78]. This has not changed the fact that cerebral MRI currently has no place in the diagnosis of post-traumatic encephalic lesions in the acute phase, as it is more time-consuming and costly to perform than CT.

2.4. Radiography of the cervical spine

X-rays of the spine should be carried out systematically in comatose head trauma patients and should reveal the cervico-dorsal hinge and the upper cervical spine in search of associated spinal lesions [67].In conscious trauma patients, this examination is guided by the functional signs described, such as localised spinal pain, a vicious posture, or radicular symptoms in the upper limbs [66].

VI. Progressive forms of HED in PCF

FCP HEDs are classified either according to their evolutionary pattern, which makes it possible to individualise three acute, sub-acute and chronic forms, or according to the duration of the free interval.According to the evolutionary mode, acute forms are those diagnosed and treated within the first 24 hours after the trauma, subacute forms are those that appear between the 2nd and 7th day after the trauma and chronic forms are those that appear after the 7th day [78,79]. Lecuire et al [79] define progressive forms according to the free interval, distinguishing between superacute forms with a free interval of less than 6 hours, acute forms with a free interval of between 6 and 24 hours, subacute forms with a free interval of between 24 hours and 7 days and chronic forms with a free interval of between 7 days and several months.

1. High-acuity forms

None of our patients presented with this type of sudden onset. The free interval is short (less than 06 hours), and these are the most serious forms, as they can result in a deep coma immediately after a violent TC. However, in general, it is after a short free interval of barely a few hours that a coma rapidly develops, with respiratory problems and sometimes signs of decerebration, without the presence of signs of localised bleeding of arterial origin, and there are often associated parenchymal lesions. Overall mortality is therefore very high [79]. Toshiaki Hayashi et al [14] found acute HED of the PCF in 14 patients (66.66%).

2. Acute forms

Acute forms represent the most classic and most frequent form of the disease. Although potentially serious, these forms give us a better chance of intervening, as the symptoms develop after an interval.They represented 45% in the series by Thierry [11] and 48.8% in the series by Edson Bor-Seng-Shu [21]. Altay Sencer et al [28] reported that 31 patients presented with an acute form, i.e. 77.5% of cases. Aykut Karasu et al [20] reported 59 out of 65, or 90%, and A. Kabre et al [13] found 9 acute forms out of 20 patients studied, or 45%.

The occipital point of impact and the notion of ICP may guide the diagnosis. During the free interval, the patient may present with occipital headaches, posing a problem of differential diagnosis with upper cervical spine disorders. These headaches may be accompanied by vomiting, which is strongly suggestive of an intracranial lesion. Signs of localisation may appear at the same time as disturbances of consciousness, but can be misleading. Finally, paralysis of the cranial nerves and papilledema are usually only visible in the terminal phase. Cerebellar signs are absent or masked by consciousness disorders.]. Toshiaki Hayashi et al [14] studied 21 HEDs in PCF, only 5 patients had localised signs pointing to the presence of cerebellar oedema. towards the posterior fossa, whereas in the other patients there was no sign of specific localization of the PCF.Besson et al (58) evaluated 100 HED of PCF, 51 of which were acute forms. They found 49 patients with no cerebellar signs. In our study, we noted the acute form of HED in PCF in 11 patients (56%).

3. Subacute forms

It is these forms that most often present clinically with localised signs pointing to PCF, making diagnosis easier. Symptoms appear 2 to 7 days after the trauma. A.Kabre [13] found this form in 50% of his patients. Edson Bor-Seng-Shu et al [21] reported 18 cases of subacute forms in a series of 43 patients, i.e. 41.9% of cases. Aykut Karasu et al [20] reported 4 cases out of 65, i.e. around 6%, and Altay Sencer et al [28], in a series of 40 patients, observed 08 sub-acute forms, i.e. 20%.Classically, there is an ICP, but this may be absent and the patient may present with occipital headaches accompanied by vomiting, sometimes associated with a stiff neck which may wrongly suggest a subarachnoid haemorrhage [57,58]. Clinically, we may be able to orient ourselves towards HED of the PCF if we find the notion of an occipital point of impact, especially associated with headaches in the same region, when the stiffness of the neck is intense, of delayed onset and especially contrasting with signs of generalised hypotonia with osteotendinous hyporeflexia. Signs of localisation are of great help, namely static or kinetic cerebellar syndrome, often unilateral, isolated or associated with contralateral pyramidal syndrome [58].Attention must be paid to other signs which may have a localising value, such as incoercible rocket-like vomiting and swallowing disorders, which indicate a formidable complication - bulbar compression. These Symptoms may be associated with mixed nerve involvement and, more rarely, hypoglossal nerve involvement [57,58]. In its sub-acute form, HED of the PCF behaves like a rapidly expanding process that gradually ruptures the anchoring veins, which then help to increase its volume. Although the volume collected is moderate, even small, in the inextensible posterior cerebral fossa, the cerebellum and brainstem are rapidly repressed and compressed. Compression of V4, obstructing Luschka's and Magendie's holes, can lead to potentially serious hydrocephalus. In our study, eleven patients (80%) had subacute HED of PCF.

4. Chronic forms

No patient presented with this form of FCP HED in our work. These are the forms that appear after the 7th day of the trauma. The chronic form is rare and presents with a subtentorial expansive process with signs ofHTIC and a cerebellar syndrome with or without signs ofbrain stem involvement [49]. Venous or diploid bleeding has been suggested as an explanation for this long evolution [13].Thierry et al [11] reported 01 cases among these 20 patients; A Kabre et al [13] found this form in 5% of these patients. Edson Bor Seng-Shu et al [21] reported 4 cases of chronic forms in a series of 43 patients, i.e. 9.3%. Altay Sencer [28], in a series of 40 patients, observed a chronic form in 2.5% of cases, while Aykut Karasu [20] reported it in 2 patients out of 65, i.e. a percentage of 3%.

VII. Treatment

Extradural haematoma is an extreme neurosurgical emergency. Once the diagnosis has been made, appropriate treatment must be instituted rapidly. Contrary to what is classically described, this study shows that the number of PCF HEDs operated on has decreased over the years. In fact, the percentage of conservative treatment has increased over the years from 6.97%[21] in 2004 to 24.61% in 2008[20] and 56% in our study. This is explained by the fact that the diagnosis of HED has become earlier and the indications much more standardised thanks to the advent of cerebral CT, advances in intensive care and the rapidity of secondary transport to centres with a neurosurgical unit. The classic "exploratory trepanation" has become anecdotal and even dangerous [20,21,61].

1. Conservative treatment

Conservative treatment was recommended in 14 of our patients (56%). Numerous authors have reported cases of spontaneous resorption of HED in PCF. They agree that symptomatic treatment should be used in the absence of consciousness disorders and focal signs of cortical and/or brainstem compression.Edson Bor-Seng-Shu [21] reported 03 cases treated conservatively. Altay Sencer et al [28] and Aykut Karasu et al [20] published 11 and 16 cases respectively. Roka YB et al [15] reported a series of 43 patients, 10 of whom were treated conservatively. In the series described, one patient in Altay Sencer's series [28], four patients in Aykut Karasu's series [20], three patients in Roka YB's series [15] and 3 patients in our series required secondary surgery following an alteration in neurological status or an increase in the volume of the HED on the follow-up CT scan. According to Benmoussa [41], even greater caution is required in two specific areas: the posterior cerebral fossa and the temporal fossa. Allowing compression to develop in these areas is not harmless, and the condition may worsen, sometimes at lightning speed. For this reason, several authors have recommended rigorous clinical and scannographic criteria for the choice of conservative treatment [82- 86]:

1.1. Clinical criteria for conservative treatment

The majority of authors agree that only patients with asymptomatic HED, with a preserved state of consciousness and in the absence of any focal signs, are considered candidates for conservative treatment [82-84].

1.2. Scannographic criteria for conservative treatment

In the case of a sustentorial HED, we have retained for conservative treatment a HED whose volume is less than 30 ml, whose thickness is less than 15 mm and when the displacement of the midline is less than 5 mm [61,84]. The CT criteria for HED in the PCF are similar to those for sustentorial HED, with the exception that the volume must be less than 10 ml. A HED of 10 ml or more in the small PCF may produce the same degree of midline deviation as a HED of 30 ml in the larger supratentorial compartment [61,84].

1.3. Monitoring conservative treatment

1.3.1. Clinic

The extreme urgency of surgical intervention in the event of neurological deterioration justifies rigorous hourly clinical monitoring of all the parameters predictive of deterioration, i.e. the state of consciousness assessed using the Glasgow score (GCS), exaggeration of the signs of HTIC such as headaches and vomiting, the appearance of new signs not previously present such as irritability and dizziness, signs of cortical involvement and suffering (pupillary anomalies, motor deficit, aphasia, neck pain), respiratory distress, haemodynamic failure and neurovegetative disorders [85]. An attentive and well-informed neurosurgical team is therefore essential to ensure that a secondary surgical conversion is always possible if any of the above-mentioned parameters appear or worsen.

1.3.2. Radiological :

While the contribution of CT is important for the initial therapeutic decision. However, it is no less important for monitoring patient progress.Shetty et al [61], Almenwar SA et al [67] and Weiss N et al [84] have agreed on the importance of repeating brain CT scans during the hospital stay, even if the patient remains asymptomatic. CT can detect signs of haematoma expansion and its effect on adjacent structures, and can also detect the occurrence of complications such as hydrocephalus and tonsillar involvement [67].The most detailed possible analysis of all the CT parameters is necessary when carrying out any CT scan. Servadei [86] has proposed a practical scheme for performing follow-up CT scans in patients who have not undergone HED surgery (figure 25).

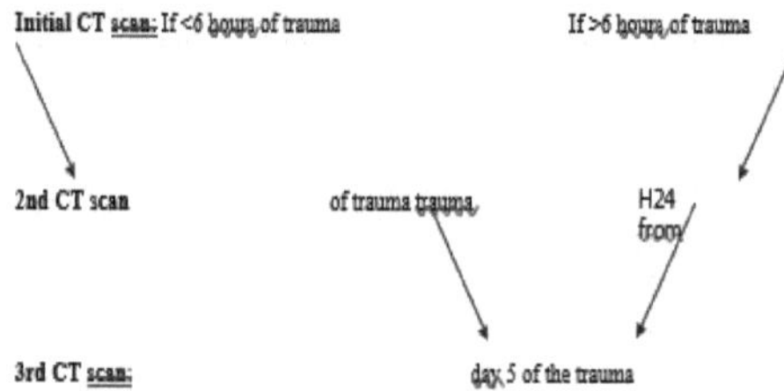

Figure 25: Time taken to perform and monitor CT scans in patients undergoing conservative treatment for HED of the PCF

Follow-up CT scans are routinely carried out even in the absence of clinical signs, and must be performed as a matter of extreme urgency as soon as any clinical sign of worsening appears.We felt that follow-up CT is of paramount importance in the surveillance of any HED in PCF.

1.3.3. Duration of surveillance

We did not find a precise consensus in the literature concerning the length of hospitalisation and therefore monitoring in patients with HED of the PCF.In recent reviews, some authors have taken the view that the patient should remain under observation until total resorption of the HED in the PCF (confirmed radiologically). However, this has resulted in a very long hospital stay (over 20 days).Servadei [86] suggested a 15-day monitoring period with repeated CT scans in order to minimise the risk of delayed neurological deterioration. Kunckey et al [87] noted that the average time to decompensation in his 7 non-operated patients was 2 to 7 days, 5 of which were within the first 24 hours, and one within the first three days. He concluded that the risk of neurological decompensation was greater during the first 24 hours and proposed an average observation period of 7 days. More recent reviews [18,28,84] have confirmed that this 7-day monitoring period is sufficient to protect most non-operated patients from the risk of secondary neurological damage.

2. Surgical treatment

2.1. Criteria for surgical treatment

2.1.1 Clinical criteria

Any HED in PCF should be evacuated urgently if the patient has presented with altered consciousness or localised neurological signs. According to the majority of authors, this is the main criterion guiding the indication for surgery [42, 44,45].

2.1.2 Radiological criteria

The indication for surgery was retained in cases of bulky HED with a thickness exceeding that of the bone opposite, in cases of significant mass effect with displacement of the midline greater than 5 mm, in cases of involvement with total or partial obliteration of the perimesencephalic cisterns and in cases of compression and displacement ofV4 [11,20,61].

2.2. The surgical technique

All our patients underwent a suboccipital craniectomy combined with a haemostasis procedure. The patient's positioning is essential: he or she must be placed in the prone position, while ensuring that the abdomen remains free of any compression to avoid venous stasis and allow good ventilation (use of cushions under the thorax and pubis and not under the abdomen). The Park-Bench position can also be used [81]. The incision was suboccipital, vertical, paramedian, and extended from the curved occipital line to the spinous process of the axis (C2). The presence of the muscle mass of the suboccipital muscles required incision of the muscle at the level of the median raphe and methodical haemostasis. The sub-occipital craniectomy is carried out with a lost bone and is extended from the foramen magnum, which is systematically opened until the lateral sinus is visualised above. If there is any doubt about the integrity of the lateral sinus, the craniectomy is stopped above the insertion of the suboccipital muscles. Haemostasis of the sinus can be achieved by tamponade and suspension of the dura mater [81].If, despite these manoeuvres, haemostasis has not been obtained, a new trepanation is carried out at a distance from the lateral sinus, completed by a craniectomy, leaving a bony bridge over the lateral sinus, over which the dura mater above and below the sinus is suspended. Thierry [11] published a case where a first trepanation had been performed in another hospital directly on a torn lateral sinus. The patient arrived in the department in a very serious condition and the team was unable to stop the haemorrhage due to the absence of a support point for the suspension, hence the importance of this technique for stopping all venous haemorrhages under good conditions. If the HED of the FCP extends to the occipital region, a supra-occipital widening of the incision and an occipital craniectomy should be envisaged, particularly in the following cases that the sustentorial HED is thick. This was the case in one of our patients who underwent evacuation of a PCF HED and an associated homolateral sustentorial HED at the same time [81]. Systematic laminectomy of the atlas (C1) remains a controversial issue, depending on the author. It allows better decompression of the PCF [11,18,20].

The next step is to perform a haemostasis procedure [82]. This procedure depends essentially on the origin of the bleeding. Bleeding from a meningeal artery can be controlled by means of a clip, ligation or simply by coagulation with bipolar forceps. If the source of the bleeding is a venous sinus, haemostasis can be achieved by applying a flap of occipital muscle and holding it in place with simple pressure. Gelatin or haemostatic matrices may be used to tamponade the wound. Finally, haemostasis can be achieved using Horsley bone wax in the event of bone bleeding [18, 20, 81]. In our series, 3 patients (37.5% of those operated on) had bleeding from the dura mater, 2 patients (25% of those operated on) had bleeding from the lateral sinus, one patient (12%) had bleeding from a bone fracture and 25% of patients had no bleeding source.Thierry et al [11] studied 20 HED of the PCF. In 4 patients, the origin of the bleeding was the posterior meningeal artery, in 9 patients, the torcular and the posterior part of the superior longitudinal sinus, and in 3 patients, the lesion resulted in bilateral detachment of the entire posterior part of the superior longitudinal sinus, the torcular and the proximal part of the lateral sinus. Kabre et al [13] also analysed 20 cases of HED of the PCF, in which the origin of the bleeding could only be found in half of the cases. In 7 cases it was the lateral sinus and in 2 other cases the venous bleeding was associated with a wound in the posterior meningeal artery; in the remaining 03 cases the haemorrhage came from the torcular.Edson Bor-Seng-Shu et al [21], out of 43 cases of HED of the PCF, found that the origin of the bleeding in only 20 patients. In 17 cases the origin was the lateral sinus and in 3 cases the bleeding was due to oozing from the meningeal vessels. Malik NK et al [60] found venous bleeding originating from the sinuses in 13 patients (27.08% of cases) and fractural bone bleeding in 7 patients (14.58%). The origin of the bleeding was not identified in 28 patients (58.33% of cases). Toshiaki Hayashi et al [14] found bleeding of arterial origin in 9.51% of cases, the lateral sinus was responsible for the bleeding in 14.28% of cases and the origin of the bleeding was the occipital sinus in 4.75% of cases.In addition, the origin of the bleeding may be mixed, arterial and venous. Thierry et al [11] published one case among 20 where a classic temporal HED fused to the posterior fossa with a fracture of the temporal scale which detached and injured the sigmoid sinus. Kabre et al [13] also published 02 cases of HED of the PCF where the origin of the bleeding was a mixed artery from both the posterior meningeal artery and the lateral sinus.

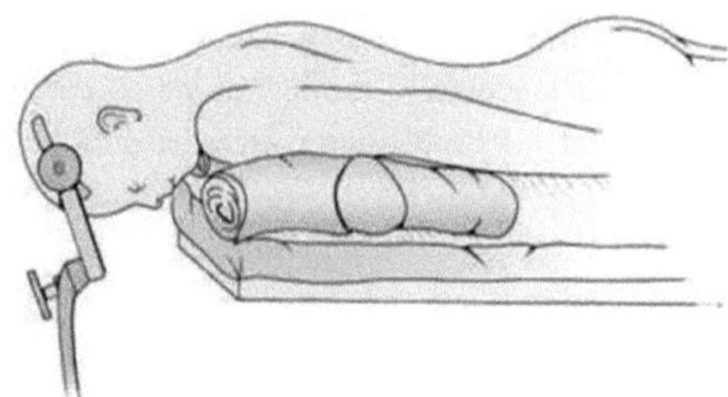

Figure 26: The prone position in neurosurgery.

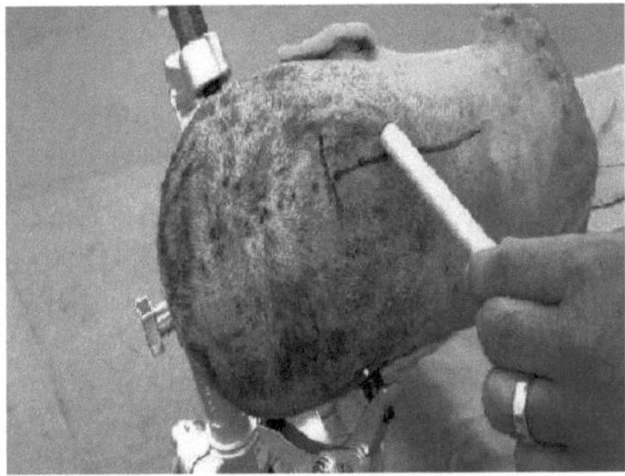

Figure 27: The suboccipital midline incision (cadaver view).

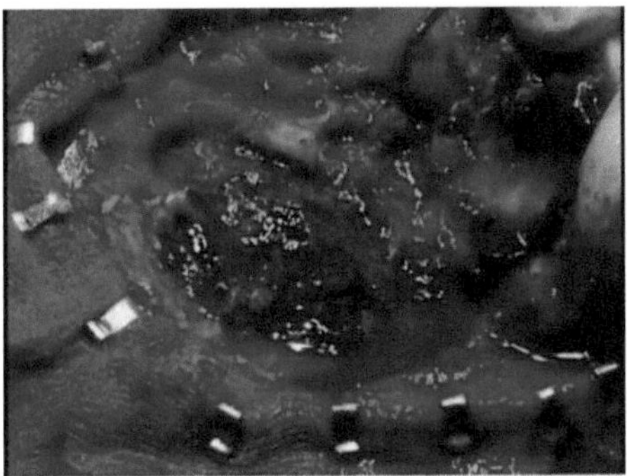

Figure 28: Operative aspect of HED of the PCF after suboccipital craniectomy.

2.3. Medical treatment

Decompressive surgery must be combined with effective neuro-resuscitation aimed at combating central and systemic brain damage (ACSOC and ACSOS) and maintaining vital functions [52].

2.3.1 Pre-operative

In the event of immediate coma, intubation and effective ventilation of the patient is imperative to combat hypoxia and hypercapnia, which are factors that aggravate brain damage. Sedation is achieved with short half-life drugs [53].Cardiovascular disturbances must be corrected and systemic arterial pressure stabilised [53,55].An overt state of shock is corrected by vascular filling, which must be limited to what is strictly necessary, to avoid hypervolaemia favouring cerebral oedema. Transfusion is necessary in the event of acute anaemia, as is the correction of any ionic disorders [53-55].Medical treatment for cerebral oedema must be initiated:

- Osmotherapy with 20% Mannitol at a dose of 0.25 to 1g/kg over 20 min, every 4-6 hours provided the patient is haemodynamically stable [55].

▪ Loop diuretics such as furosemide reduce the volume of blood and venous pressure, by lowering CSF secretion, which causes a fall in intracranial pressure. The usual dose is 20 mg IV every 06 hours [55].

▪ Fluid and sodium restriction: All injured people are subject to fluid and sodium restriction. hydro-sodium supplementation with 10 ml/kg of isotonic saline for 48 hours [55].

Simple measures can also be taken to combat cerebral oedema, such as elevating the head to 30° to improve venous drainage, and assisted hyperventilation with controlled hypocapnia [53,85].

2.3.2 Intraoperative

Transfusion should be considered whenever necessary, particularly in children, given their low blood mass; HED from PCF can lead to haemorrhagic shock. Anti-oedema treatment may be maintained [53,55].

2.3.3 Post-operative

The aim of postoperative resuscitation is to ensure rigorous clinical monitoring, maintain a good fluid and electrolyte balance, and carry out careful nursing to avoid trophic disorders. Antibiotic therapy is necessary in all cases of open head trauma [53,85].

VIII. Course and prognosis :

1. Mortality

The mortality rate for HED in PCF has been significantly reduced thanks to the advent of cerebral tomography and advances in emergency and transport services, as well as neuro-resuscitation. The outcome is closely linked to early diagnosis and treatment [49, 87, 88, 89].

Table 17: Mortality rates by author and by year.

Author	Year of publication	Total number of case	Mortality
Roda [25]	1983	83	26,5%
THIERRY [13]	1990	20	10%
Prusty [64]	1995	17	17,6%
A Kabre [13]	2001	20	5%
	2004	43	4,7%
Hayashi [14]	2007	21	4,8%
Aykut Karasu [20]	2008	65	3,8%
Roka YB [15]	2008	43	7%
Bogdan Asanin [16]	2009	18	11,11%
Jae-Won Jang [22]	2011	34	2,9%
Altay Sencer [28]	2012	40	0%
Meknassi [18]	2014	29	0%
Our series	2015	25	0%

2. Follow-up :

Patients treated for HED of the PCF should receive regular follow-up at the neurosurgery outpatient clinic, based on clinical examination and cerebral CT scan injected with iodinated contrast [89,91].There is no consensus in the literature regarding the frequency of CT scan monitoring after the end of treatment, but it is accepted that at least one CT scan of the brain without contrast injection should be performed within one month of the end of treatment. Late recurrence of HED in PCF is exceptional.Cerebral MRI can contribute to the assessment of the sequelae of head trauma [85,89].

3. After-effects

Sequelae have also become increasingly rare thanks to advances in neuro-resuscitation and neuroradiological investigations. This morbidity may be neurological, intellectual or psycho-affective [89-93].

3.1. Functional sequelae

The GOS score at three months was favourable, i.e. between 4 and 5 in 23 of our patients, in line with most of the literature reviews (table 18).

Table 18: Patient trends by series

Author	GOS between 4 and 5	GOS between 2and 3	GOS at 1
A Kabre [13]	80%	15%	5%
Edson Bor-Seng-Shu [21]	90,6%	4,6%	4,7%
Toshiaki Hayashi [14]	85,5%	9,5%	4,8%
Aykut Karasu [20]	92,4%	3,8%	3,8%
Meknassi [18]	93,1	6,9%	0%
Our series	92%	8%	0%

Despite this often satisfactory "neurological" outcome, the family and socio-professional reintegration of people with cranial trauma is not a simple matter.

3.2. Subjective brain injury syndrome

Subjective head injury syndrome or post-concussion syndrome is defined as the set of disorders experienced by injured people who have suffered a concussion and who have non-objectifiable symptoms [90].It occurs in 50-80% of cases. Symptoms are dominated by headaches, dizziness and hearing or visual problems. Symptomatic drug treatments are often disappointing in these patients [90,93].

3.3. Neuropsychological consequences

They mainly concern memory function.In most cases, the disorders are very discreet, resulting in learning and memory disorders [90,91].In children, these after-effects are relatively mild, but attention and memory can be inhibited to some extent, leading to failure at school. These sequelae accompany all post-traumatic deficit states. Character disorders (mood instability, impulsivity), emotional regression and demands on the family are a constant feature. These sequelae depend in part on the family's overprotective reaction (which avoids any risk or initiative for the child, thus preventing timely reintegration into social life), or excessively demanding reaction (which requires the sometimes handicapped individual to make an effort that is clearly beyond his or her strength, at least temporarily) [89, 92, 93].

CONCLUSIONS

Extradural haematoma (EDH) or epidural haematoma is an uncommon but potentially serious complication of cranial trauma. It is defined by the accumulation of blood in the epidural space, i.e. between the internal table of the bone and the dura mater. It represents the neurosurgical emergency par excellence.It occurs very rarely in the posterior cerebral fossa, but is particularly serious because it is usually the result of direct, violent trauma applied directly to the occipital region.The aim of our study was to describe the current management of extradural haematomas of the posterior cerebral fossa.The management of extradural haematomas has benefited greatly from advances in medical imaging, and in particular from the advent of cerebral computed tomography (CT), which not only makes it possible to carry out a complete emergency assessment of the lesion, but also to establish the indication for surgery, and to monitor and follow up patients after treatment.We studied the management of extradural haematomas of the posterior cerebral fossa by the neurosurgery department of the Military Hospital of Tunis concerning 25 patients over a period of 16 years (January 2000 to December 2015). We included all cases of extradural haematomas of the posterior cerebral fossa whose diagnosis was confirmed by cerebral CT. Patients with supratentorial HED isolated on cerebral CT were excluded from our study.We studied the epidemioclinical and radiological data, therapeutic attitudes, monitoring methods and outcome, comparing our results with those of other published series.We found an annual frequency of 1.56 cases per year, with an average age of 26.84 and a predominance of males, with a sex ratio of 3.16. Aetiologies were dominated by road traffic accidents (48%), followed by domestic accidents (28%) and assaults (24%). The mechanism of trauma was direct impact on the nucho-occipital region in 76% of our patients.The average consultation time was 24.08 hours, the notion of initial loss of consciousness (PIC) was found in 76% of cases and the free interval was found in 56% of cases. Clinical signs were dominated by intracranial hypertension, present in 88% of patients.Assessment of the state of consciousness using the Glasgow score showed that 88% of our patients had a GCS of between 13 and 15, 8% of patients had a GCS of between 8 and 12 and 4% of our patients had a GCS of less than or equal to 7. Focal neurological signs were present in 48% of cases, dominated by cerebellar syndrome (40%) and meningeal signs (16%).We noted that 20% of our patients had an occipital scalp wound and that all our patients were haemodynamically and respiratorily stable.All patients underwent an emergency cerebral CT scan without injection of contrast medium. The diagnosis of extradural haematoma of the posterior cerebral fossa was established in all our patients. FCP HEDs were all unilateral, with 64% on the right side and 36% on the left. The typical spontaneously hyperdense biconvex lens appearance was noted in 80% of cases. The thickness of the HED was greater than 10 mm in 32% of cases, with a mass effect.CT scans also revealed an occipital fracture line in 60% of patients and enabled us to identify other cranioencephalic lesions in 52% of patients, including supratentorial HED in 12% of cases. Extracranial lesions were found in 24% of our patients, dominated by facial lesions (16%). Surgical treatment was carried out as an emergency in 8 cases, i.e. 32% of cases. It was undertaken secondarily in 3 patients (12%), following a secondary alteration in the state of consciousness or following a follow-up cerebral CT scan showing an increase in the volume of the HED of the PCF. All patients underwent a suboccipital bone-through craniectomy with evacuation of the haematoma and haemostasis.Only one patient (4%) underwent a supratentorial flap during the same operation, allowing evacuation of a homolateral sustentorial HED.We determined the origin of the bleeding in 6 patients, i.e. 75% of those operated on and 24% of the population as a whole. The bleeding was duarterial in 3 patients, a lateral sinus wound was found in 2 patients and the bleeding was of bony origin, fractured in only one patient. With regard to postoperative monitoring, all patients underwent clinical monitoring for signs of HTIC and GCS on a twice-daily basis, with a complete neurological examination every day to look for signs of localisation.In our series, 14 patients benefited from conservative treatment, i.e. strict clinical and scannographic monitoring combined with medical treatment consisting of measures to combat factors of cerebral aggression of central origin (HTIC, cerebral oedema and hydrocephalus), and of systemic origin by maintaining effective ventilation, a stable haemodynamic state, and the correction of any ionic disorders or anaemia. All our patients underwent a follow-up cerebral CT scan without injection of contrast medium 24 to 48 hours after evacuation of the haematoma. In 100% of cases, we found a significant reduction in the thickness of the HED to ≤ 5mm, or even its disappearance, associated with complete regression of the mass effect.Subjects who did not undergo surgery initially had a follow-up cerebral CT scan every 24 to 48 hours for the first 5 days. This showed a slight increase in the size of the haematoma in 3 cases, which did not require surgery. However, the increase in the size of the haematoma wasin 3 patients, requiring surgical evacuation. During the follow-up of patients at the neurosurgery outpatient clinic, over a period of 6 months to 2 years,4 patients were lost to follow-up and 72% of the remaining patients received at least 2 consultations and a follow-up brain CT scan in the 3 months following discharge.

The outcome was favourable in 92% of cases.

We can therefore conclude from the various data studied in the literature and from our own series that extradural haematoma of the posterior cerebral fossa is a rare pathology but represents a genuine diagnostic and therapeutic emergency, which may be life-threatening and cause serious neurological sequelae. Its management requires close collaboration between the neurosurgeon and the intensive care physician.

Road accidents are the main cause.

The clinical picture of HED in PCF is classically defined by a three-stage drama, beginning with the trauma, which may be accompanied by an initial loss of consciousness, followed by a period of lucidity or free interval, and then the secondary aggravation phase, in which neurological signs and altered consciousness appear.However, the typical clinical form of extradural haematoma of the posterior cerebral fossa is not always present, and the presence of a point of impact in the cervico-occipital region and a notion of a free interval should raise the diagnosis.Its association with other intracranial lesions, as well as with extracranial lesions in the context of polytrauma, must always be carefully assessed, given the risk of lesion potentiation. Cerebral CT without injection of contrast medium is the key examination, making it possible to establish the diagnosis as a matter of urgency, to complete the lesion assessment and to guide therapeutic management.Conservative treatment may be proposed if the patient is perfectly conscious with a normal neurological examination and if the thickness of the haematoma is less than 15mm with a volume of less than 10 ml, with no mass effect on the median structures.In other cases, the treatment for extradural haematoma of the posterior cerebral fossa is essentially surgical, consisting of a suboccipital craniectomy combined with opening of the foramen magnum, evacuation of the haematoma and haemostasis.In addition, surgical treatment is required in the event of secondary deterioration in the state of consciousness, or the appearance or worsening of signs of intracranial hypertension, whether or not associated with signs of localisation. On CT, an increase in the thickness of the haematoma or in the mass effect, or the appearance of threatening hydrocephalus, also requires surgery.Lastly, the medical treatment consists of measures to combat the factors that can lead to cerebral damage of central origin (HTIC, cerebral oedema and hydrocephalus), and of systemic origin by maintaining effective ventilation, a stable haemodynamic state and the correction of any ionic disorders or anaemia. Clinical and scannographic monitoring is essential, particularly in the absence of surgery, given the possible worsening which would require urgent surgical evacuation, but also in patients who have undergone surgery, in order to assess the quality of evacuation of the haematoma, as well as the degree of progression of associated cerebral and/or cerebellar lesions.The overall prognosis for extradural haematomas of the posterior cerebral fossa is good, with death occurring only in forms seen late, in forms with profound impairment of consciousness and in forms associated with other intracranial or extracranial lesions forming part of a polytrauma.Tonsillar involvement and obstructive hydrocephalus due to V4 compression are the most serious complications, and most often fatal. The functional after-effects are mainly represented by the subjective syndrome of head trauma and the neuropsychological after-effects, which can affect the patient's quality of life even after discharge from hospital and have a major impact on most of their daily activities.

REFERENCES

1. Brown AW, Elovic EP, Kothari S, Flangan SR, Kwasnica C. Congenital and acquired brain injury: epidemiology, pathophysiology, prognosis, innovative treatments, and prevention. Arch Phys Med Rehabil. 2008;89Suppl1:S3-S8.
2. Maas AL, Stocchetti N, Bullock R. Moderate and severe traumatic brain injury in adults. The Lancet Neurology. 2008;7:728-41.
3. Bouchet A, Guilleret J. Anatomie topographique descriptive et fonctionnelle, le système nerveux central. 6th edition.Paris: SIMEP;1991.

4. Albert L, Rhoton JR. Cerebellum and fourth ventricle. Neurosurgery.2000;47:7- 27.

5. Standring S. Gray's anatomy, the anatomical basis of clinical practice. 39th edition. London. Elsevier;2008.
6. Singh A, Aaron P, Wessell BS, Vijay K, Anand M, FACST et al.Surgical anatomy and physiology for the skull base surgeon.Operative Techniques in Otolaryngology- Head and Neck Surgery. 2011;22(3):184-93.
7. Chirag RP, Juan C, Fernandez M,Wei-Hsin W, Eric W, Wang M et al.Skull base anatomy. Otolaryngologic Clinics of North America. 2016;49(1):9-20.
8. Albert L, Rhoton JR. Cerebellar arteries. Neurosurgery. 2000;47:29-68.

9. Chapman PR, Asim K, BagR, Tubbs S, Gohlke P. Practical Anatomy of the Central Skull Base Region.Seminars in Ultrasound, CT and MRI. 2013;34(5):381-92.

10. Albert L, Rhoton JR. Posterior fossa veins. Neurosurgery. 2000;47:69-92

11. Thierry A, Sauteaux JL, Chandan N, Marin D, Giroux M. Extradural haematoma of the PCF. Neurochirurgie. 1990;36(1):39-44.
12. Costa Clara JM, Clavaimunt E, Ley L, Lafuente J. Traumatic extradural hematomas of the posterior fossa. Childs Nery.Syst. 1996;12(3):14-8.
13. AKabre, Alliez JR, Kaya JM, Bou Harb G, Reynier Y, Alliez B et al. Extradural haematoma of the posterior fossa. Neurochirurgie.2001;47:105-10.
14. Hayashi T, Kameyana M, Imoizumi S, Kamii H, Onuma T. Acute epidural hematoma of the posterior fossa - cases of the acute clinical deterioration. American Journal of Emergency Medicine. 2007;25:989-95.

15. Roka YB, Kumar P, Bista P, Sharma GR, Adhikari D. Traumatic Posterior Fossa Extradural Haematoma.Nepal Med Assoc. 2008;47(172):174-8.
16. Bogdan Asanin. Traumatic epidural hematomas in posterior Cranial Fossa.Acta clin croat. 2009;48:27-30.

17. Cuirea AV , Nuteanu L, Simionescu U, Georgescu S. Posterior fossa extradural hematomas in children, report of nine cases. Childs Nerukyst. 1993;9(4):224-8.

18. Meknassi Mohamed. les hématomes extraduraux de la fosse cerebrale posterieure(a propos

de 29 cas et revue de la litterature) [Thesis]. Medicine :Fès; 2014.131p.

19. Dirim BV, Öruk C, Erdogan C, Gelal F, Uluç E. Traumatic posterior fossa hematomas. Diagn Interv Radiol. 2005;11:14-18.
20. Karasu A , Sabanci PA, Izgi N, Imer M, Sencer A, Cansever T et al. Traumatic epidural hematomas of the posterior cranial fossa.Surgical Neurology. 2008;69:247- 52.
21. Bor-Seng-Shu E, Aguiar PH, De Almeida Leme RJ, Mandel Almir Ferreira De Andrade M, Marino R. Epidural hematomas of the posterior cranial fossa. Neurosurg Focus. 2004;16(2):1-4.

22. Jang JW, Lee JK, Seo BR, Kim SH. Traumatic epidural haematoma of the posterior cranial fossa. British Journal of Neurosurgery. 2011;25(1):55-61.
23. Besson G,Legu Yader J, Bagot D'Arc M, Garre H. HED of the FCP. Diagnostic problems (10 observations). Neurochirurgie. 1978;24:53-63.

24. Zuccarello M, Andrioli GC, Fiore DL, Longatti PL, Pardatscher K, Zampieri P. Traumatic posterior fossa hemorrhage in children. Actat Neurichir. 1982;62(2):79- 85.

25. Roda JM, Gimenez D, Perez-Higueras A, Blazquez MG, Perez Alvarez M. Posterior fossa epidural hematomas: a review and synthesis. Surg. Neurol. 1983;5:419-24.

26. Jamjoom A, Cummu SB, Jamjoom ZA. Clinical characteristics of traumatic extradural hematoma: a comparison between children and adults. Neurosurg. 1994;17(4):277-81.
27. Ersalin Y, Mutluer S. Posterior fossa extradural hematomas in children. Pediatr. Neurosurg 1993;19(1):31-3.

28. Sencer A, Aras Y, Osma N Akcakaya M, Goker B, Krisis T et al. Posterior fossa epidural hematomas in children: clinical experience with 40 cases. J Neurosurg Pediatrics. 2012;9:139-43.

29. Ammirati M, TomitaT. Posterior fossa epidural hematoma during childhoud. Neurosurgery. 1984;14:541-4.
30. Sautreaux JL, Binnert D, Thierry A, Pelikan MC, Ordas M, Couaillier JF et al. CT scanning in cranial traumatology, critical study of 500 cases. Neurosurgery. 2000;28:263-70.

31. Belotti C, Medina M, Baralle S, Oliveri G, Et-Torre F, Suturiale C et al. Chronic extradural hematomas of the posterior cranial fossa. Surg neurol. 1987;27:580-4.

32. Sheng HS, Youb CG, Yang L, Zhang N, Lin J, Lin FC et al.Trephination mini-craniectomy for traumatic posterior fossa epidural hematomas in selected pediatric patients. Chinese Journal of Taumatology. 2017;20(4):212-5

33. Cook RJ, Dorsch NWC, Fearnside MR, Chaseling R. Outcome prediction in extradural haematomas. Acta Neurochirurgica. 1988;95:90-4.
34. Jamieson KG, Yelland JDN. Extradural hematoma: report of 167 cases. J. Neurosurg. 1968 ;29:13-23.

35. Remond J, Fisher G. Hématome extradural, sous dural, intracérébral : dg et principes du traitement. Rev Prat. 1990 ;40(26):2495-8.

36. Servadei F, Faccani G, roccella P, Seracchioli A, Godano U, Ghadirpour R et al. Asymptomatic extradural haematomas. Results of a multicenter study of 158 cases in minor head injury. Acta Neurochir. 1989;96(1-2):39-45.

37. Jiang JY. Head trauma in China.Injury.2013;44(11):1453-7.

38. Rabbai O, Hachimi A, Charra B, Benslama A, Motaouakkil S. Extradural haematoma of the vertex due to rupture of the superior longitudinal sinus. Annales françaises d'anesthésie et de réanimation 2006;25:462-70.

39. Devaux B, Roux FX, Chodkiewicz JF. HED in the era of the SAMU and the scanner. Neurochir. 1986;32:221-5.

40. Willis J, Kiessling IV, Dean A. Hertzler II, Drucker DEM, Heather S et al.Traumatic Frontal Epidural Hematoma Caused by Multiple Arterial Injuries in the Anterior Fossa.World Neurosurgery. 2017;97:757-8.

41. Benmoussa H, Mouhoub F, Tamehmacht M, Rifi L, Bellakhdar F. Non-operated extradural haematoma. A propos de 3 observations. Neurochirurgie. 1992;38:42-45.

42. Sakai H, Takagi H, Ohtaka H, Tanabe T, Ohwada T, Yada K. Serial changes in acute extradural hematoma size and associated changes in level on consciousness and intracranial pressure. J Neurosurg. 1988;68:566-70.

43. Chen TY, Wong CW, Chang CN, Lui TN, Cheng WC, Tsai MD et al. The expectant treatment of "asymptomatic" supratentorial epidural hematomas.Neurosurgery. 2013;32(2):176-9.

44. Pang D, Horton JA, Herron JM, Wilberger JE, Vries JK. Nonsurgical management of extradural hematomas in children.J Neurosurg. 1983;59:958-971.

45. Tuncer R, Kazan S, Ucar T, Acikbas C, Saveren M. Conservative management of epidural hematomas: prospective study of 15 cases. Acta Neurochir. 1993;121:48- 52.

46. Kaufman HH, Herschberger J, Koptnik T, Mc Allister P, Hogg J, Conner T et al. Chronic extradural haematomas: indications for surgery. Br J Neurosurg. 1992;6:359- 64.

47. Aoki N. Rapid resolution of acute epidural hematoma. J Neurosurgery. 1998;68:149-151.

48. Nixon M, Ambekar S, Zhang S, Markham C, Akbarian-Tefaghi H, Morrow K et al. Traumatic Injury to the Posterior Fossa.2014;32(4):943-55.

49. Nagi S, Ben Reguiga M, Kaddour C, Miaoui A, Ghorbel D, Maatallah Y et al. Extradural hematoma of the posterior fossa: A propos de 4 pediatric observations. Journal de Pédiatrie et de puériculture. 2007;20:29-32.

50. Kumar R, Kataria R, Sardana V, Gupta P.Post-traumatic retroclival epidural hematoma with atlantoaxial dislocation: A rare case report and review of literature. 2014;11(2):154-8

51. Paul E. Marik L, Varon J,Trask T.Management of head trauma.Chest. 2002; 122:699-711.

52. Tavender EJ, Bosch M, Green S, O'Conner D, Pitt V, Phillips K et al. Quality and consistency ofguidelines for the management of mild traumatic brain injury in theemergency department. Acad Emerg Med. 2011;18:880-9.
53. Pearson J, Henning J, Woods K. Management of major trauma. Anaesthesia & Intensive Care Medicine. 2017;18(8):383-5.
54. Teasdale G, Jennett B. Assessment of coma and impaired consciousness.A practical scale.Lancet.1974;2:81-4.
55. Vrankovic DJ, Splavski B, Hecimovic I. Acute traumatic hematomasof the posterior fossa: experience with eleven cases. Neurol Croat. 1994;43:21-30.
56. Wynell-Mayow W, Guevel B, Quansah B, O'Leary R, Carrothers AD. Cambridge Polytrauma Pathway: Are we making appropriately guided decisions?.Injury. 2016;47(10):2117-21.
57. Cataltepe O, Ozcan OE. Traumatic epidural haematomaof the posterior fossa in childhood: 16 new cases anda review of the literature. Br J Neurosurg.2003;17:226- 9.

58. Oxford RG, Chesnut RM. Neurosurgical Considerations in Craniofacial Trauma. Facial Plastic Surgery Clinics of North America. 2017;25(4):479-91.
59. Wintermark M, Sanelli PC, Anzai Y, Tsiouris AJ, Whitlow CT. Imagingevidence and recommendations for traumatic brain injury:conventional neuroimaging techniques. J Am Coll Radiol. 2015;12:1-14.
60. Malik NK, Makhdoomi R, Indira B, Shankar S, Sastry K. Posterior fossa extradural hematoma: our experience and review of the literature. Surgical Neurology. 2007;68(2):155-8.
61. Shetty VS, Reis MN, Aulino JM, Berger KL, Broder J, Choudhri AF et al. ACR Appropriateness Criteria Head Trauma. 2016; 13(6):668-79.
62. Garza Mercado R. Extradural hematoma of the posterior cranial fossa report of seven cases with survival. J Neurosurg.1983;59(4):664-72.

63. Rincon S, Gupta R, Ptak T. Chapter 22 - Imaging of head trauma. Handbook of Clinical Neurology. 2016;135:447-77.

64. Prusty GK, Mohanty A. Posterior fossa extradural hematoma. J Indian Med Assoc. 1995;93(7):25-8.

65. Salcman M, Pevsner PH. The value of MRI in head injury-comparison with CT. Neurochirurgie.1992 ;38:329-32.
66. Miller JD, Murray LS, Teasdale GM. Development of a traumatic intracranial hematoma after a "minor" head injury. Neurosurg. 1990;27(5):669-73.

67. Almenawer SA, Bogza I, Yarascavitch B, Sne N, Farrokhyar F, Murty N et al. The value of scheduled repeat cranial computed tomography after mild head injury: single- center series and meta-analysis. Neurosurgery. 2013;72(1):56-64.

68. Hounsfild G N. Picture quality of computed tomography. Am J Roentgenol. 1976;127:3-9.

69. Metting Z, A Rödiger L, De Keyser K, van der Naalt J. Structural and functional neuroimaging in mild to moderate head injury. The Lancet Neurology.2007;6:699- 710.

70. Mathis JM, Sowers JJ, Zelenik ME. Pathognomonic CT findings of posterior fossa epidural hematoms.Comput radiol. 1984;8:395-401.
71. Smith HK, Miller JD. The danger of ultra-early computed tomographic scan in a patient with an evolving acute epidural hematoma. Neurosurgery. 1991;29:258-60.

72. Ford LE, Mc Laurin RL. Mechanisms of extradural hematomas. 1963;20:760-769.
73. Servadei F, Nanni A, Nasi MT, Zappi D, Vergoni G, Giuliani G et al. Evolving brain lesions in the first 12 hours after head injury: analysis of 37 comatose patients. Neurosurgery.1995;37:899-906.
74. Poon WS, Rehman SU, Poon CY, Li AK. Traumatic extradural hematoma of delayed onset is not a rarity. Neurosurgery. 1992;30:681-6.

75. Fankhauser F, Uske A, De Tribolet N. Delayed epidural haematomas: a case report of 8 patients. Neurochir. 1983;29:255-60.

76. Mathis JM, Sowers JJ, Zelenik ME.Pathognomonic ct findings of posterior fossa epidural hematomas.Computerized Radiology. 1984;8(6):395-401.

77. Kurosu A, Amano K, Kubo O, Himuro H, Nagao T, Akihiro A et al. Clivus epidural hematoma case report. J. Neuro. Surg.1990;72(4):660-2.
78. Orrison WW, Gentry LR, Stimac GK, Tarrel RM, Espinosa MC, Cobb LC. Blinded comparison of cranial CT and MR in closed head injury evaluation.AJNR AM J Neuroradiol. 1994;15(2):351-6.
79. Lecuire J, Hor F, Bret PH, Deruty F, Capoeville. la scannographie d'urgence dans les hématomes extraduraux intracrâniens traumatiques. Lyon chirurgia, 1983;79(1):3- 4

80. D'Avella D, Servadei F, Scerrati M. Traumatic intracerebellarhemorrhages: a clinico radiological analysis of 81 cases. Neurosurgery. 2002;50:16-25.

81. Paillas J, Lecuire J. Nouveau traité de technique chirurgicale. Paris: Masson;1975.
82. Lahat E, Livne M, Barr J, Schiffer J, Eshel G.The management of epidural hematomas-surgical versus conservative treatment.Eur J Pediatr. 1994;153:198- 201.

83. Moura Dos Santos AL, Plese JPP, Ciquinic O, Shu EBS, Manreza LA, Marino R et al. Extradural hematomas in children. Pediatr Neurosurg. 2004;21:50-4.
84. Sullivan TP, Jeffrey G, Jarvik W, Cohen A. Follow-up of conservatively managed epidural hematomas: implications for timing of repeat CT. AJNR Am J Neuroradiol. 1999;20:107-13.

85. Weiss N, Galanaud D, Carpentier A, De Montcel ST, Naccache L, CoriatP et al. A combined clinical and MRI approach for outcome assessment of traumatic head injury for comatose patients. J Neurol. 2008;255:217-23.
86. Servadei F, Faccani G, Roccella P, Seracchioli A, Godano U,Ghadirpour R et al. Asymptomatic extradural haematomas.Results of a multicenter study of 158 cases in minor head injury.Acta Neurochir. 1989;96(1-2):39-45.

87. Knuckey NW, Gelbard S, Epstein MH. The management of "asymptomatic" epidural heamatomas.A prospective study.J Neurosurg. 1999;70:392-6.

88. Pozzati E, Tognetti F, Gavallo M, Acciarri N. Extradural hematomas of the posterior cranial fossa: observation on a serie of 32 consecutive cases treated after the introduction of computed tomography scanning.Surgical Neurology. 1989;32(4):300-3.

89. Kuday C, Uzan M, Hanci M.Statistical analysis of the factors affecting the outcome of extraduralhematomas: 115 cases. Acta Neurochir. 1994;131(3-4):203-6.

90. Wester K. Decompressive surgery for "pure" epidural hematomas: does neurosurgical expertise improve the outcome?.Neurosurg. 1999;44(3):495-500.

91. Servadei F. Prognostic factors in severely head injured adult patients with epidural hematomas. Acta Neurochir. 1997;139(4):237-8.

92. Karasawa H, Furuya H, Naito H. Acute hydrocephalus in posterior fossa injury. J Neurosurg. 1997;86:629-32.

93. Suresh HS, Praharaj SS, Indira Devi B, Shukla D, Sastry Kolluri VR. Prognosis in children with head injury: an analysis of 340 patients. Neurology India. 2003;51(1):16- 8.

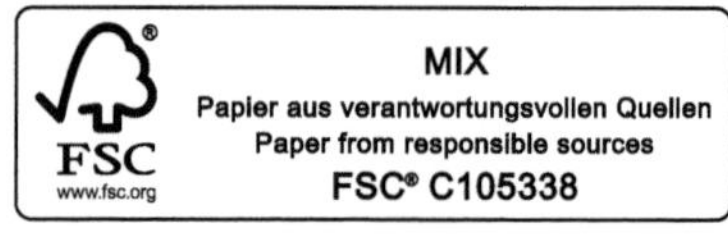

Printed by Books on Demand GmbH, Norderstedt / Germany